Cluster Headaches & Tension Headaches.

Managing Pain The Natural Way.

Cluster Headaches & Tension Headaches:
Causes, Remedies, Relief, Symptoms,
Treatment, Managing Pain, Exercises all
included

by

By Robert R

Table of Contents

Foreword

No one will fully understand the feeling of a cluster headache unless you have had the misfortune to experience them. Likewise, no one will fully understand the effects of living with tension type headaches that can occur day in and day out.

With these conditions, diagnosis can often be slow and the sometimes daily headaches can have a devastating effect on a person and affect every aspect of their life.

While there are many medications that are available to help manage these two conditions more effectively and to help improve the quality of a patient's life, this book goes beyond that and has been written with the aim of helping explore all of the possible treatments out there.

As well as outlining the medical approach to treating cluster headaches and tension type headaches, this book's main focus is to concentrate on the many effective methods of relieving pain naturally.

Several experts have contributed to this book so that the patient can be clear on what to expect from each of the natural therapies suggested, and while the book does focus on the natural pain relieving benefits of alternative remedies, it does not advocate these remedies over any other treatment; the aim is to enable patients to learn how to use natural treatments alongside their current treatment regimen, where suitable.

As cluster headaches and tension type headaches are often misunderstood, and the major problems caused by them often go unreported, it is hoped that this book will go a long way towards enhancing the understanding of the various treatments out there. The book also aims to help patients suffering from either of these conditions to avoid any of the possible triggers for these debilitating illnesses, and offers practical approaches to managing them more effectively.

The book will also share patients' experiences with these conditions and provide hints and tips that they use to alleviate their suffering and how to treat a cluster headache effectively.

Introduction

Everyone experiences headaches at some point during their life. However, for some of us, the pain can become a weekly or daily experience and begin to impinge on a person's quality of life.

Even when a patient isn't living with the pain of a cluster headache or a tension type headache, they can begin to live in fear of when the next one is going to occur and, unfortunately, there are no cures for cluster headaches.

While headaches might seem like a minor ailment to some, they can have a devastating impact on people's lives, affecting their ability to work, to socialise or to participate fully in the activities they once enjoyed.

This book will begin by focusing on the symptoms and the treatments available for headache sufferers and will detail the signs and symptoms of tension headaches and cluster headaches.

However, as many people do not like the idea of being on long term pain medication, and some are often reluctant to take prescribed medications because of the potential side effects, this book will explore the numerous natural methods that are available for treating the symptoms of tension headaches and cluster headaches.

However, these therapies should not be used without consulting with a GP/consultant/physician first as they will be able to best advise you if there is a chance that any of the treatments might interact with any of the medications or treatments that you are currently undergoing.

This book is aimed at showing that there are plenty of natural treatment options available and as they normally don't have any side effects, these natural therapies are a safe way to help manage symptoms.

As well as detailing therapies such as acupuncture, nutrition and homeopathy, this book will help the reader to make the lifestyle changes that are often needed to defeat or manage their pain.

Statistics

According to figures from the World Health Organization, 47% of the global population is affected by headaches. Tension Type Headaches (TTH) affect up to 3% of the population and these types of headaches often begin in the teenage years; more women than men are affected.

If the TTH are episodic they will often last for a few hours, however, they can also last several days. Chronic TTH can have a debilitating effect on a patient, and the attacks can be unrelenting.

Cluster headaches are much less common and it is estimated that they affect 1 in every 1000. They are more common in men than they are in women.

People who develop cluster headaches will usually be in their twenties and they have both episodic and chronic forms.

Many patients will experience a considerable delay between the onset of their symptoms and being diagnosed. The average time before a patient is diagnosed can be as long as five years.

Cluster headaches often have a severe impact on everyday life and up to 20% of sufferers will have to give up their work due to their symptoms.

Chapter 1) Different Types of Headaches

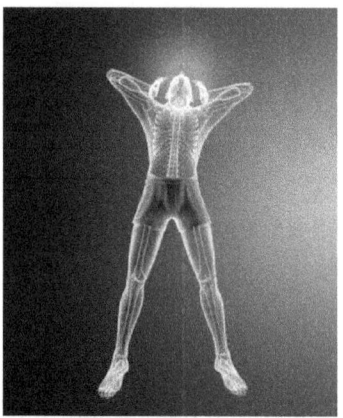

While this book largely focuses on the natural treatments available for cluster headaches and tension headaches, this section of the book will give an overview of the different types of head pain that people can experience and detail their symptoms.

1) Different Types of Headaches

There are several different types of headaches and all of them have different causes and factors that will contribute to them. However, headaches can be divided into two categories: primary headaches and secondary headaches.

Primary headaches include cluster headaches, tension-type headaches or tension headaches, and migraines. With primary headaches, there is no underlying medical condition that causes them.

Secondary headaches are related to another medical disorder. For example, patients with high blood pressure, an injury or a nerve condition such as neuralgia can all experience headaches. The cause of chronic headaches will be different for every patient.

2) What Causes Headaches?

The branches of the trigeminal nerve carry sensations to the head and neck area. It is when a nerve ending, known as a nociceptor, is exposed to a headache trigger such as stress, that the trigeminal nerve will send a message to the thalamus. The thalamus gland will then carry a pain message to the brain, triggering a headache.

Detailed in the following section are some of the most common types of headache. If a patient has constant headaches or if they are uncertain as to the cause of a headache, then they should seek medical advice

3) Common Types of Headaches

a) Medication Related Headaches/Rebound Headaches

People who regularly take painkilling medication can go on to develop medication related headaches or rebound headaches. This is quite common in patients who take Paracetomol and anti-inflammatory drugs such as Ibuprofen, and other over-the-counter drugs. Prescribed pain killing medications can also have the same effects.

If a patient is taking drugs such as anti-inflammatory medications to help manage their symptoms and they notice that they are getting headaches more frequently, or that the headaches are more severe than they were previously, then the patient should talk about this with their GP or consultant to discuss alternative forms of medication.

b) Sinus Headaches

Sinus problems often occur after a cold and they are one of the common causes of headaches. However, in some patients, sinus problems can become constant and this can cause constant sinus headaches, face pain, congestion, pain or headache behind the eyes, and a general feeling of being under the weather.

c) Sinus Headache – Treatment

Conventional treatment usually centres on the prescription of antibiotics if it is believed that there is an infection. It might also be suggested that the patient uses decongestant tablets or sprays. However, these types of medications are only suitable for short term use and if they are used long term, then they can make the congestion worse.

Many patients with sinus headaches find that regular steaming can help to reduce the feeling of pressure around the head and face. To enhance the effects of this, add some drops of eucalyptus essential oil to the water and breathe in the vapour until the feeling of pressure begins to fade. Steaming regularly can also help to reduce tension in the head area.

d) Chronic Daily Headaches

One of the causes of constant headaches is known as chronic daily headaches. They can sometimes be triggered by illness, but sometimes there isn't a known cause.

Chronic headache treatment usually consists of medication such as antispasmodics or anti-depressants.

e) Vascular Headaches

Migraines are vascular in their nature and cause symptoms such as sensitivity to light, sensitivity to sound, visual disturbances, nausea and vomiting. The pain caused by migraines can often be enough to make a person cry and these types of severe headaches can have a huge impact on the quality of a person's life.

Patients can also experience migraines without aura, which means they don't get visual disturbances such as flashing lights prior to the migraine.

There are also silent migraines. This means that a patient will experience all of the symptoms associated with a migraine such as nausea, sensitivity to light and sound and visual disturbances but they won't get a headache.

As with cluster headaches, migraines can have numerous triggers and these will all vary from person to person. Sometimes it is food or alcohol, for other people it is stress. Women can also be prone to migraines before their period; menstrual migraines are quite common.

Food can also be a trigger when it comes to a migraine. Foods that cause headaches/migraines include chocolate, cheese, foods with excess salt and some additives.

Cluster Headaches

Chapter 2) Cluster Headaches

1) What are Cluster Headaches?

Cluster headaches strike one side of the head. These headaches cause severe pain and they come in "clusters" so a patient might have series of cluster headaches that can happen every day – sometimes several times a day – and the attacks can sometimes last for weeks.

The pain from severe cluster headaches is often felt behind one eye and the eye might also become swollen. Some patients also get a runny nose during an attack and other patients experience nausea.

During a cluster headache, some patients might have an increase in their blood pressure and heart rate.

The pain from these headaches is so bad that one patient described having a desire to jump from a window while experiencing a cluster headache as the pain was so severe.

Some patients will get migraine-like symptoms preceding a cluster headache and they might experience an aura – or visual disturbance before the attack. The attacks come in "clusters" and the patient can go pain free for weeks and months before experiencing another series of cluster headaches.

Cluster headaches can sometimes be hereditary and they can sometimes be the result of a head injury.

2) The Difference between Cluster, Tension Headaches and Migraine

Although some of the symptoms of cluster headaches can be the same as migraines, there are some defining factors that make cluster headaches different from migraines.

The major differences are the intensity of the pain caused by cluster headaches and the frequency of them. A migraine will usually last a day or two and the pain can be extremely intense, but after that the pain tends to go. However, as one cluster headache sufferer explains, "A cluster headache will hit you with a pain that is unequal to any pain I have ever felt. It will hit you fast and when it leaves it leaves you worrying when it will be back and finally it hits you repeatedly".

Some patients can experience seven or more attacks throughout the day and such is the intensity of the pain, some sufferers call them "suicide headaches".

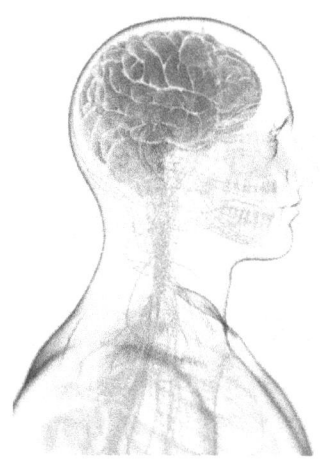

3) Symptoms of Cluster Headaches

Symptoms of a cluster headache can be similar to those of migraines; however, the intensity of a cluster headache is far worse than that experienced by migraine sufferers.

The symptoms of a cluster headache include:

- A stuffy or blocked nose
- Severe eye pain
- A feeling of pressure in the head
- Pulsating pain in the face
- Problems with vision
- Sensitivity to light
- Sensitivity to sound
- Loss of consciousness
- Yawning

After an attack a patient can feel groggy and drained.

3) What causes Cluster Headaches?

There are a number of different causes of cluster headaches. These triggers will vary from person to person, but here is a list of some of the common triggers.

The triggers for cluster headache, including food and drink:

- Osmophobia (strong smells – petrol diesel, perfume (cheap spirit based ones), paint, nail varnish etc.
- Photophobia (bright lights)
- Extreme heat (not a good idea to be a chef!)
- Extreme cold (not a good idea to be a polar explorer or lover of snow!)
- Phonophobia (loud noise)
- Sleeping in the daytime

- Violent exercise (particularly if it raises body temperature)
- Alcohol, (for some even in sherry trifle, or liquor gateaux). NB One exception to alcohol in food is where the alcohol has been cooked out, as in Coq au Vin.
- It is also a good idea to stay away from hot curries as these can act as a trigger in some people. If you like curry, then choose a milder version rather than ones that are too hot.

4) Cluster Headaches – Diagnosis

Cluster headaches are usually diagnosed once the patient has described the symptoms to their GP or consultant. Sometimes further tests might be carried out, but often these are not deemed necessary if the doctor or consultant is sure of the diagnosis.

Chapter 3) Medications and Treatments for Cluster Headaches

Treatment for cluster headaches often involves triptan based medication. Sometimes a medication might be prescribed in conjunction with another one; this will all depend on the severity of the symptoms. Medication for cluster headaches will also help to prevent some attacks, but it won't eliminate them completely. The best treatment for cluster headaches will vary from patient to patient. These are some of the medications commonly prescribed for the treatment for a cluster headache.

1) Sumatriptan

Triptan based medications are commonly prescribed for helping patients to manage the pain of a cluster headache.

Triptans in their tablet form are not strong enough to prevent a cluster headache so they are often given as a spray. In addition, triptans, when given in tablet form, take too long to work, because they first need to be absorbed by the gut before they can begin to work. However, triptans can be a useful medication to be taken at night time to provide pain relief throughout the night.

Val from the Organisation for the Understanding of Cluster Headaches (OUCH) explains the various forms of triptans to help treat cluster headaches:

"These medications come under various brand names some of them are:Imigran injections (subcutaneous sumatriptan); Imigran tablets (sumatriptan tablets);Imigran nasal sprays (sumatriptan nasal spray); Migard (Frovatriptan); Zomig (zolmitriptan nasal spray and tablets).

"Migard or Frovatriptan Migard has a half-life of up to 26 hours in the body, and is useful for days when you really could do without an attack, such as a wedding, a presentation at work, an examination etc. I use them to get me through long-haul flights. We tried using them as a regular preventive (off-label use) but we found that the pain free period got shorter and shorter until it wasn't worth using it."

Sumatriptan and Frovatriptan are also used to help treat migraine attacks. Sumatriptan is available in an over-the-counter medication in the form of Imagram Recovery. However, as explained on the previous page, these are not suitable for cluster headaches.

Side Effects:

Frovatriptan also has a number of side effects, although not everyone will experience them. Some of the side effects of this kind of medication include a dry mouth, digestive problems, chest pains and a feeling of being overtired.

Any patients who are bothered by their side effects should talk to their doctor about them.

Side effects of triptans can also include dizziness, feelings of nausea, feelings of weakness and muscle pain.

2) Prednisone

Prednisone is a corticosteroid and it is often used to treat inflammatory conditions as well as diseases such as multiple sclerosis. It is also prescribed as a treatment for cluster headaches.

Prednisone is often only prescribed for short periods of time and will sometimes be prescribed alongside another form of medication. When a patient needs to come off Prednisone, then the doctor will reduce the dosage over a period of time so that the patient doesn't suffer any undue side effects.

If it is deemed necessary that Prednisone needs to be given longer term, then the dosage prescribed will be low.

Side Effects:

As with all medications there are some side effects with taking Prednisone and these will vary from patient to patient. However, one common side effect is feeling hungry all of the time and some patients gain weight while on this medication.

3) Verapamil and Cluster Headaches

Verapamil is another medication that is often prescribed for the treatment of cluster headaches.

The medication is taken three times a day. Verapamil can be an extremely effective method of managing cluster headaches and some say that this form of medication has saved their lives. Verapamil can play an important role in cluster headache prevention and patients who take this medication often report fewer attacks.

Side Effects:

However, there are also some side effects that can come with Verapamil such as dizziness, tiredness, irregular heartbeat, itching, skin rash and numbness, etc. Many patients agree that this type of medication is worth sticking with, as even with some of the side effects, their symptoms are much easier to manage.

Some patients are lucky enough to not experience any problems while on this medication. If anyone has side effects that are intolerable then they should speak to their doctor or consultant about trying a different medication.

4) Lidocaine Nasal Spray

Lidocaine comes in several different forms, but it is often given as a nasal spray for the treatment of cluster headaches.

Lidocaine is prescribed for migraine sufferers as well as patients with cluster headaches. It is used for treating cluster headaches and acts quickly. However, it is not entirely understood how Lidocaine works. Nasal sprays containing Lidocaine are available to buy over the counter, however, they should not be used without talking to a doctor first.

Side Effects

There are several side effects associated with Lidocaine. These can include dizziness, skin sensitivity and changes in the heart rate.

5) Oxygen for Cluster Headaches

Oxygen is often used to help patients with cluster headaches. It is not certain how oxygen alleviates symptoms. However, as the Organisation for the Understanding of Cluster Headaches (OUCH) explains:

"The exact mechanism of oxygen working is not known, but many sufferers start to yawn heavily prior to attacks, an indication that the brain lacks oxygen – a wrong message sent out by the hypothalamus perhaps – so inhalation of high flow oxygen reverses that message."

6) Melatonin and Cluster Headaches

It is believed that melatonin, the hormone produced by the pineal gland, plays a role in the development of cluster headaches. Melatonin has been shown to successfully treat patients with chronic cluster headache and episodic cluster headaches.

There is more information on Melatonin in the second part of the book.

Chapter 4) Natural Treatments for Cluster Headaches

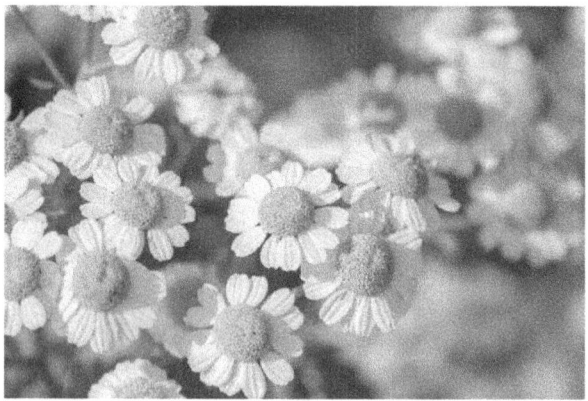

Medications are the main management tools for patients with cluster headaches; however, many patients like to try natural approaches. If, as a sufferer of cluster headaches, you decide to try natural methods of reducing the symptoms, then speak to your care team first to ensure that there won't be any contraindications with any of the medication that you have been prescribed.

Unfortunately, there are few natural remedies for cluster headaches and the options for home remedies for cluster headaches are limited, such is the intensity of the pain. However, some patients say that they experience an improvement in their symptoms when taking certain supplements, but there is little in the way of scientific evidence to back this up and more research needs to be done.

Detailed below are some suggested natural cluster headaches remedies that have shown promise for the treatment of cluster headaches.

1) Feverfew

Some patients have found that feverfew can help to reduce the symptoms of cluster headaches. The herb is well known to be helpful to patients suffering from migraines as well.

Feverfew has been shown to reduce symptoms such as nausea and vomiting and it can also limit the spasms that occur in the vascular system.

Capsule forms of feverfew are available. However, feverfew is easy to grow and some people like to cultivate their own and add feverfew to their meals, for instance, adding some of the leaves to a sandwich. However, for most people it is a better idea to buy a standardized product.

Contraindications:

The herb should not be taken by children, pregnant women or those on blood thinning drugs.

2) Vitamins and Minerals for Cluster Headaches

There are some vitamin therapy regimens that are used by cluster headache sufferers, however these have yet to be approved for use in the UK and they are currently only being trialed in the United States.

However, there is limited evidence to suggest that some vitamins and minerals can be effective at reducing the frequency of cluster headaches. Detailed in this chapter are some vitamins and minerals that cluster headache sufferers have found useful. However, they won't work for everyone. In addition, there is also evidence that some people with cluster headaches might be deficient in some vitamins/minerals and some supplements are known to reduce pain. Some of these supplements are detailed here. However, they are not suggestions for treatment and should not be tried without first speaking to the person responsible for your care.

a) Vitamin B2

B2 could be one of the natural remedies for cluster headaches, according to research.

Studies have shown that patients who supplement their diet with vitamin B2 have fewer cluster headache attacks. It is recommended that 400mg of vitamin B2 or riboflavin is taken every day to help lessen the number of cluster headaches.

Vitamin B2 can also be obtained from foods such as meat, cheese, breads, cereals and bananas.

If supplementing with B2, make sure that you take a B complex vitamin as well to avoid depleting the levels of other essential B vitamins.

Contraindications:

There are several types of medications such as anti-depressants, Luminal and Benemid that can interact with B2 supplements.

b) Magnesium

Magnesium is a mineral that has been found to be helpful for patients with cluster headaches. Some patients with cluster headaches have been found to have low levels of magnesium and this mineral is also useful to patients with tension type headaches as it helps to relax tight, tense muscles.

For people who don't want to supplement with magnesium, try adding plenty of nuts, seeds, and green vegetables to the diet.

Magnesium is best taken in a supplement that also contains calcium and boron. It is important to take magnesium and calcium at the correct ratio and boron is essential for enabling the proper absorption of magnesium, so buying a supplement that contains all three minerals is best.

Another option is to try a magnesium spray. These are designed for use at night to enable people to get a good night's sleep. However, the sprays can also be used throughout the day whenever the muscles can be felt tightening and tensing up.

c) DLPA

DLPA or DL-Phenylalanine is an amino acid that has been shown to act as a natural pain reliever and there is some evidence to suggest that it could be helpful for patients with cluster headaches. This amino acid has also been shown to help lift the mood and also plays an important role in brain function.

DLPA can be brought in supplement form or, to increase the amount of this amino acid, try adding more high quality protein foods to the diet. DLPA can be found in meat, eggs and fish and other high protein foods.

d) Vitamin D3

Taking vitamin D3 to help reduce the symptoms of cluster headaches is something that is currently being trialed in the States. However, this involves giving large amounts of the vitamin, and this is not something that people should be attempting on their own.

Many people do report a reduction of symptoms when supplementing with D3, but this should not be tried without consultation with a doctor first as the effects of taking vitamin D3 in excessive doses still aren't known.

In addition to the above suggestions, Alison Wyndham, founder of the Wyndham Centres in Baldock and London, has worked as a physiotherapist since the 1970s and in the 1980s she qualified in alternative therapies. During her career, Alison Wyndham has often treated patients with cluster headaches and tension headaches.

Alison Wyndham has the following advice on natural therapies that people might find helpful for managing both cluster headaches and tension headaches.

3) Natural Supplements

– Willow Bark has been used for many years to reduce pain. Its active ingredient is salicin which is metabolised in the human body into salicylic acid.

– B3 in the nicotinic acid (niacin) form is a vaso dilator. It will cause a 'blushing' sensation and increased heat and can often help a headache in the early stages.

– B6, B12 and folic acid have been known to reduce the severity and frequency of headaches, by reducing the levels of homocysteine, an amino acid derived from the normal breakdown of proteins in the body. Too much in the blood can lead to inflammation and damage to the arterial walls.

– SerraEzyme a proteolytic enzyme that works as a natural anti-inflammatory and pain reliever. This should not be taken with blood thinning drugs.

4) Physiotherapy – invariably tension headaches are caused by muscle tightness in the neck and treating the neck with mobilisations and deep muscle work can be helpful.

Our aim is to mobilise the joints, improve posture, loosen and stretch the tight muscles and encourage the correct muscle function.

5) Dental – if you have had your wisdom teeth removed it can change your bite, which will create muscle tightness around the jaw, face and neck, which in turn can cause headaches. It is worth seeing an orthodontist specialising in bites to check it is in the correct position.

6) Food Allergies

I have found that 80% of tension or cluster headaches are caused by food sensitivities and by taking out of the diet the offending foods, it can make a huge difference.

7) The Alexander Technique

The Alexander technique teaches that use affects functioning. If we misuse ourselves with bad posture, stiffening our neck muscles and altering the position of our head, hunching our shoulders or holding our breath, these bad patterns cause muscle imbalances that can lead to headaches. By learning how to prevent these bad patterns we can restore our natural poise and become pain free.

Chapter 5) Chinese Medicine

The Chinese Medical Treatment Approach to Tension Headaches and Cluster Headaches by the AcuMedic Clinic

During its development over the past 5,000 years, Chinese Medicine has established a detailed framework for diagnosing and treating various types of headaches, including tension and cluster headaches, with acupuncture and Chinese herbs.

1) Introduction

Chinese Medicine classifies headaches according to the syndromes (the root cause) behind the pain. A syndrome is established by identifying the time of the headache's onset (day, evening or during sleep at night); its duration and location in the head; the character of the pain (e.g. dull or sharp, throbbing or distending) and which factors (rest, food) ameliorate or aggravate the headache, as well as which emotions might trigger the headache.

Once the syndrome which describes the root cause of headache has been established through diagnosis, Chinese Medicine uses acupuncture and herbal medicine to treat the patient. The principal approach to treatment is to treat the root cause of the symptom (headache), with the relief in pain being a natural outcome of the treatment.

Based on information gathered during diagnosis, the Chinese Medical doctor can determine if the headache is of an external or internal origin. Frequent external causes are cold and hot wind while internal causes (which are more common) come in two types: empty type (e.g. shortage of body's essential energy in the body or lifeblood) and full type (e.g. excess dampness or phlegm in the body; stagnation in the circulation of lifeblood). Based on this detailed information and identification of the syndrome identified during diagnosis, acupuncture points and Chinese herbs are selected to the treat the patient's headache.

2) Chinese Medicine and Cluster Headaches – Treatment and Diagnosis

Cluster headaches are of the full type and of internal cause which usually tends to be 'Liver-Yang Rising'. This is the name of the syndrome which refers to the process whereby an excess in the body's hot energy (Yang – the opposite of Yin) is flowing upwards through the channel which links the liver with the head. Such uprising of energy agitates the body and causes painful heat inside the head.

Cluster headaches can be treated by identifying the root cause of the Liver-Yang Rising syndrome. The possible root causes are: a shortage of blood within the liver; a shortage of cooling energy (Yin – the opposite of hot Yang) within the liver or within both liver and kidneys; or, a shortage of Yin in the liver or kidneys combined with a shortage of Yang within the kidneys.

The basic principle behind Chinese Medical treatment of cluster headaches is to use certain acupuncture points and Chinese herbs that can control the uprising flow of hot energy, calm the liver and, depending on the root cause of Liver-Yang Rising identified in the patient, replenish and nourish the blood and cooling energy within the liver and/or kidneys.

At this point it should become clear that in Chinese Medicine the treatment is always patient-centred in the sense that it is individualised to the patient's personal needs so that the person is treated and not merely his or her symptoms. For example, two patients suffering from identical symptoms of tension headache might receive different Chinese Medical treatments with different acupuncture points and Chinese herbs selected for each patient.

Chapter 6) Diet and Cluster Headaches

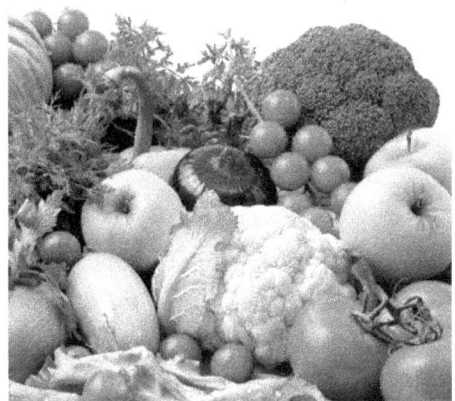

Many patients with cluster headaches say that certain foods will trigger their headaches. Some patients say that once they have excluded some foods or ingredients from their diet, their symptoms have improved considerably. Other patients suffering from cluster headaches have found that once they stop drinking alcohol, then their symptoms begin to improve and they have fewer cluster headaches.

However, there is little in the way of scientific evidence to suggest that certain foods can trigger cluster headaches and the experts say that it is a coincidence that when these people have cut out certain foods or ingredients, their symptoms have improved.

If diet is an area you want to explore, this chapter will detail some of the foods and ingredients that cluster headache patients believe contribute to their symptoms.

However, it is not a good idea to start eliminating food without taking medical advice. When a person is unwell, they need all of the nutrition that their body can get so eliminating foods is not ideal as it can leave the patient devoid of certain nutrients. Before changing your diet, speak to a doctor first.

Here is a list of some of the foods that nutrition experts suggest avoiding, or cutting down on:

- Milk products
- Sweets
- Sugar
- Nuts
- Cold drinks (especially ice cold drinks)
- Protein Powders
- Liquor
- Wine

1) Artificial Sweeteners

Some patients with cluster headaches cite artificial sweeteners as one of the ingredients that can trigger an attack Artificial sweeteners have been associated with headaches – especially migraines – in the past. However, any evidence to suggest that there could be a link between sweeteners and headaches has so far only been anecdotal, and studies that have been carried out to establish a link, have been limited to small groups of people.

There are some cluster headache sufferers who say that as soon as they have stopped consuming foods and drink that contains artificial sweeteners, they stop getting cluster headaches. However, this may just be coincidental and there is little in the way of firm evidence to support this.

In December 2013, the European Food Safety Authority issued a full risk assessment of artificial sweeteners, including aspartame, which has often been associated with headaches. It was concluded that the sweetener was safe to consume at the current levels.

2) Nitrates

Nitrates are a form of food preservative that is often added to meats such as bacon and hot dogs. Some patients say that their headaches are worse if they consume foods containing nitrates and that consuming nitrates or nitric acid can trigger an attack.

Nitrates are known to widen the blood vessels and this is perhaps why they can trigger an attack in some patients.

3) MSG

MSG or Monosodium Glutamate is often used to add flavouring to foods. It is commonly found in products such as soy sauce and some patients with cluster headaches say that they believe that MSG can trigger an attack.

4) Preservatives

Some patients with chronic cluster headaches find that various preservatives can cause an attack.

5) Dairy/Journal Keeping

Dairy or journal keeping is an ideal way to track what you have been doing at any given time and many patients with cluster headaches find that writing down the details of the medication they are on, the foods they eat, and the stress they are under, can help them to discover patterns that might be causing or contributing to their cluster headaches.

In addition, make sure you detail the time of day, how frequently the headaches occur, and the types of medications that you are taking. Recording all of this information will help to highlight any patterns that might occur and it will give you a better idea of how to treat cluster headaches when they occur.

It is also a good idea to record all of the cluster headache treatments and detail how long they keep you pain free for, so that you can get a real ideal of how effective your cluster headache medication is in helping you to cope with your symptoms.

Chapter 7) Acupuncture for Headaches

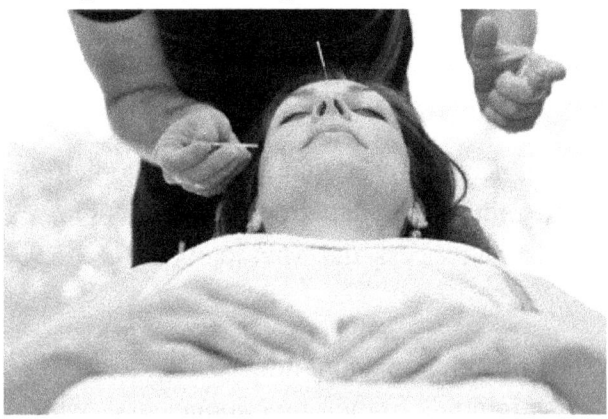

Acupuncture has been shown to be an effective treatment for both cluster and tension headaches; it has been shown to reduce both the intensity and frequency. Acupuncture is recommended by the National Institute of Clinical Excellence (NICE), the UK body that offers independent advice on the most effective ways to treat and prevent disease, as a treatment for patients suffering from headaches and some doctors recommend acupuncture for cluster headaches.

Acupuncture is an effective method of relief for many people. However, this form of treatment is not for everybody and some will respond differently from others, but many patients swear by the benefits of this kind of therapy and some have found acupuncture to provide an effective form of pain relief.

1) Side Effects of Acupuncture

Side effects from this kind of therapy are rare, but some patients might experience problems such as a minor bruising around the site of the needle, which is usually quick to heal. Some patients also experience dizziness following a treatment while some patients report feeling tired after a session of acupuncture, but overall the experience is a relaxing one.

Some patients experience a feeling of lightheadedness, but this doesn't occur with most patients. It is also advisable to eat something light before undergoing an acupuncture session.

As the prospect of having needles inserted into the skin to help alleviate their symptoms might seem daunting to some people, this next section explains the process and what to expect at a treatment session.

If a patient has any specific concern about undergoing acupuncture then they should talk to their practitioner first, who will be able to help ease any concerns ahead of the treatment.

2) Acupuncture Treatment

Ahead of the treatment the practitioner will ask a set of questions. Some of them might sound a bit random, but this is because the practitioner is trying to establish where the energy flow is blocked.

The way acupuncture is used will vary from patient to patient as each practitioner will have their own methods and they will need to take into account the individual's medical history. Although many people don't like the thought of the needles, it is not a painful process, but if the patient feels any discomfort, the practitioner will change the positioning of the needle.

Although each practitioner will have their own particular way of treating headaches depending on the symptoms the patient is suffering, the acupuncture needles will usually be placed on the meridian points of the ear, the body, or the head. Once the patient has answered a set of questions, the practitioner will have a much better idea of the symptoms and, based on this information, they will place the needles on the appropriate meridian line to help improve energy flow.

Before the session can go ahead, patients will have to first consent to the treatment and before consenting to acupuncture, the practitioner will explain all of the measures that will need to be taken to ensure that the treatment can be carried out safely.

Sessions usually last an hour, although the first session will often be longer as you'll need to go through your medical history and details of your symptoms.

Patients often don't experience an improvement in their condition straight away and it may take 3-4 sessions before noticing an improvement in the symptoms. For some patients, it might take longer and some practitioners recommend at least ten sessions before a patient can expect to witness an improvement in their condition.

3) How Acupuncture Works

Acupuncturists believe in qi and they believe that qi flows through the meridian lines of the body. When the chi or energy becomes blocked, it can lead to pain and disease. By inserting needles on specific points on the meridian lines, it is believed that it will release the block in the energy thus reducing pain and disease.

Acupuncture also acts to increase circulation and blood flow. This type of therapy is aimed at treating the underlying causes of pain such as headaches, which will often be different in each individual patient.

4) How Acupuncture Helps Headache Sufferers

Acupuncture can help headache sufferers in several ways; principally, it will help the patient to relax. People who suffer from tension type headaches and cluster headaches often carry a lot of tension in their bodies and acupuncture can allow a person to manage stress.

Using acupuncture can also help to relieve the pain of headaches and many people who undergo this form of therapy say that acupuncture has helped to significantly improve their quality of life.

Chapter 8) Managing Cluster Headaches

Medications can go a long way to helping patients better manage their symptoms. However there are a few more tools available that can help to manage cluster headaches effectively.

Some patients with cluster headaches find it useful to keep a record of the times and dates of their attacks and the types of medication that they are taking. Patients might also like to detail the symptoms of a cluster headache so that they can learn to spot the early signs and any of the cluster headache treatments that they are currently prescribed and how effective they are.

To make this easier, Christopher Delage has created an app to make managing cluster headaches easier.

The app has been made available as a free tool and can be used to record details such as the time and the intensity of the attack, the medication taken, how long the attacks last etc., and what the patient has done to bring relief for cluster headaches and their symptoms. By detailing all of the information the patient knows what to do for cluster headaches the next time they experience one.

Christopher Delage suffers from cluster headaches himself and uses the app to help manage them. It is available for android phones and can be downloaded free from the Google app store by going to:
https://play.google.com/store/apps/details?id=eu.monavf.android.monavf

Another way cluster headache sufferers can help to manage their pain is by sharing their experiences with other people who understand fully what the headaches feel like and the pain that they go through.

While talking to other patients might not tell you how to stop cluster headaches completely, there is plenty of advice available on social media sites and it can be accessed by following other people who have to deal with the symptoms of these intensely painful headaches.

One cluster headache sufferer, Julian Yates, has set up @clusterheads on Twitter so that people can share their personal experiences and exchange hints and tips.

You can read more about Julian Yates and his personal experience of cluster headaches in the next chapter.

Chapter 9) Cluster Headaches: A Personal Experience

Julian Yates, from Wells, Somerset, UK is a cluster headache sufferer & creator and host of @Clusterheads. Here, Julian shares his personal experience of cluster headaches.

"I was diagnosed with Cluster Headache in spring 2012 after six years of suffering a misdiagnosis.

"For most of those six years I was prescribed antibiotics for Sinusitis. Naturally this didn't work so I treated myself with Paracetamol and Codeine. This would kill the pain of an attack after about 1.5 to 2 hours after a dose. Unknown to me the Cluster headache attacks were ending themselves at those times so the tablets were of no help because they took too long to work."

1) Diagnosis of Cluster Headaches

"In 2012 I went back to my doctor's surgery but this time I saw a different doctor, who, after me describing my symptoms & experiences, said that he thought I may suffer from Cluster Headaches. He described CH as a neurological disease and advised that there is no real treatment, but there are ways to abort an attack. He also said that he had never seen a patient with Cluster Headache in his career and doubted any of my previous Doctors would have either, hence the 6 year delay in diagnosis.

"The diagnosis was provided following my description of pain and symptoms. The attacks would happen for periods of around eight weeks and these periods would usually happen twice a year. Attacks would normally wake me up an hour or so after I fell to sleep and last for up to two hours.

"The pain is excruciating; on the same side of my head/face every time and pain through my left temple, behind my left eye, down my left jaw and across the left side of the roof of my mouth. My left nostril would also become painful and congested. At first I thought I had a tumour in my head or a brain haemorrhage. I couldn't sit still. I paced the room banging my hand on my head. I would fall to my knees in pain rocking backwards and forwards. Nothing would stop the pain. After about 1.5 or 2 hours, all of a sudden and out of the blue the pain would just vanish as quickly as it started and I would just sit there, exhausted."

2) Treatment of Cluster Headaches

"My Doctor advised that high flow rate oxygen was NHS (National Health Service) abortive of choice and or Sumatriptan injections; however these medications were expensive so he recommended Sumatriptan nasal spray to use when an attack starts. At first the spray seemed to work, but as time went on it seemed that the time it was taking to abort the attacks was taking longer. I revisited the doctor and asked for the injections. I only took one injection. It killed the pain in minutes which was excellent, but I experienced some weird feeling in my head and chest, so I didn't take any more. It was then that I managed to convince my Doctor to agree to me using oxygen. O_2 starts to reduce the pain level as soon as I start using it and in most cases the pain is gone in 20 minutes. If after 20 minutes the pain remains, then I revert to the nasal spray. I now have 4 full standing oxygen cylinders at home and 3 ambulatory cylinders to take out with me to work etc.

3) Support

"Cluster Headache is a very lonely condition. I had never heard of it before. The worst thing that people say is that they often get headaches or migraines, but they have no idea what the pain of

Cluster Headaches is. It was because I wanted to share my experience with someone else who had the condition that I set up a Twitter account called Clustermeetingplace, @Clusterheads. After my first tweet people started to follow. These people were and are other Cluster headache sufferers and supporters of Cluster Headache sufferers. We often Tweet at midnight after attacks, share our pain, experiences, tips and support each other when feeling low. I am really proud that I set up @Clusterheads knowing that maybe I have helped someone in some little way that may improve their life."

4) Cluster Headaches – A Personal Story: Number Two

Richard Eason has suffered from cluster headaches for more than a decade. It was seven years before Richard was diagnosed and he would often suffer from up to seven attacks a day.

After being prescribed different types of medications and undergoing surgery, because the doctor's couldn't determine what was causing the symptoms, Richard was finally diagnosed with cluster headaches.

In this next section, Richard explains how he manages his symptoms and explains practical tips that will hopefully serve to help other sufferers.

"I will usually get what I call a prequel which is like a mini attack before the real headache starts."

5) Symptoms of Cluster Headaches

"This will usually start with my nose feeling stuffy or even blocked on right hand side this will cause me to rub pinch and even squash my nose as it continues to irritate me. Then I will start to get a dull ache in the right eye which will progress to feel like really bad eye strain. At this point I know a full attack is coming so I will try lying on my left hand side to relieve the pressure in my head and nose, I will also try to re-hydrate myself by drinking lots of water; this has worked on occasion but is not a fool proof counter measure.

"If a full attack occurs the symptoms above get exponentially worse. My nose will feel so blocked and pressurized that I have, on occasion, wanted to stick objects up there to ease the pain and pressure. The already painful eye ache has now progressed to a pain that is hard to describe; it feels like your eye is on fire and at the back of the eye something is stabbing at it. Now as well as this I will feel pressure between the eye and nose and a pulsating pain that will cover roughly a quarter of my face on the right hand side including the temple; the temple will become sensitive to the touch.

"The pain will become so intense that I find it hard to talk. My vision will become impaired and I will stagger to whatever hiding place I can get to. A cool dark place is usually best as I become more sensitive to light, sound and temperatures.

"At the peak of worse attacks, I will lose consciousness, which is probably for the best. I will regain consciousness at the back end of the attack feeling groggy drained and worn out."

6) Medications

Richard is treated with Verapamil tablets. The tablets are taken three times a day, and Richard explained that while some people do have side effects when taking this form of medication, he hasn't suffered any himself.

Richard says that while Verapamil is not a cure it has "massively" reduced the frequency of the attacks. He has been taking the medication for three years and says that Verapamil has given him a new lease of life.

7) Remedies for Cluster Headaches

Every sufferer of cluster headaches will have found their own ways of managing their symptoms. Here, Richard explains the methods he uses to make his cluster headache attacks easier.

"When an attack starts, drink an ice cold can of coke quickly and try to burp through nose. I don't know how it works it just does; I personally have aborted attacks with this remedy.

"Decongestants like Lemsip or hay fever medications can help some but not me personally.

"Co-codamol dissolvable 500mg tablets: inhale while tablets are dissolving. This helps to cool the inside of nose and stop it drying out, then drink water. This has not stopped attacks but has helped them to pass much quicker."

Tension Headaches

Introduction – Tension Headaches

The first part of this book focused on cluster headaches and their causes, symptoms and treatments. This next section will concentrate on tension headaches and detail ways to effectively manage the symptoms as well as detailing preventive measures that anyone can take to limit the chances of developing tension headaches.

The first few chapters will detail the symptoms, the cause of tension headaches and the medical treatment for tension headaches; and the next part of the book will explain how lifestyle changes, finding effective stress relief measures, and taking basic steps can help to reduce the occurrence of tension headaches.

As this book is largely about finding natural pain relief methods, there are also chapters on finding natural methods of treatment for tension headaches such as aromatherapy and osteopathy, in order to help the patient find the therapy that is most suitable for them and to help the reader to discover the best treatment for tension headaches.

People suffering from tension headaches can also learn about beneficial herbs, vitamins, minerals and how good nutrition can help to reduce the symptoms of tension headaches. In addition, readers can find out about natural headache remedies, tension headache remedies and advice on how to relieve tension headaches.

Once you have finished reading this part of the book, you'll know how to treat a tension headache, the cause of headaches and how to stop a tension headache. You'll also learn tips on dealing with chronic tension as well as discovering some useful tension headache home remedies and how to avoid tension headaches.

Readers will also find out how to spot the signs of a tension headache, how to tell if you have a tension headache or migraine, and find details on the treatment for chronic tension headaches.

However, as these therapies are only meant to be used as a complementary form of treatment then they should not be tried without first talking to the person responsible for your care.

Chapter 10) What are Tension Headaches?

Tension headaches or tension type headaches usually occur when the muscles in the neck and head contract. Tension headaches come in two different forms and can either be episodic or chronic.

How Long Do Tension Headaches Last?

The length of time a tension headache will last varies. For some people, the pain might last for just a few hours, while with others they can last a few days. Others might find that they feel like they have a constant headache. People suffering from frequent tension headaches should see a doctor, if they haven't already.

1) Tension Headaches -Symptoms

The symptoms of a tension headache will vary in intensity from person to person. However, there are some typical symptoms of a tension headache.

a) Chronic Tension Headache – Symptoms

Chronic tension headaches have the same symptoms as tension type headaches; however, they will be experienced more often. A patient will be described as having chronic tension headaches if they have them for fifteen days of the month or more.

Often patients can start to feel as though they have constant headaches, and tiredness can also be another common symptom of this condition.

b) Episodic Tension Headaches

Patients who have less than 15 attacks of tension headaches would be described as suffering from episodic tension headaches.

c) Where Are Tension Headaches Located?

When a patient experiences symptoms of a tension headache, they will experience problems with sleeping and a dull pain that affects both sides of the head. Signs of a tension headache also include a feeling of tension in and around the scalp area and some patients describe the pain as a vice-like feeling. Patients with tension headaches will often experience depression. Depression and headaches are often associated.

Some patients feel as though they have a constant dull headache, and this can severely affect the patient's quality of life. If a patient feels as though they have a constant tension headache then they must address all of the factors that could be causing it.

Pain in the neck can also be another common tension headache symptom as can pain in the shoulder region.

d) Tension Headaches and Dizziness

It is not uncommon for patients with tension headaches to also experience dizziness, and this can be one of the most unpleasant symptoms of a tension headache. Tension headaches and nausea are also common.

One of the contributing factors to dizziness can be tight neck muscles. There are some tips to reduce neck tension later on in the book.

e) The Difference Between Tension Headaches and Migraines

Tension type headaches and migraines can seem similar in many ways as patients will often experience symptoms such as sensitivity to light and sound. However, patients with tension headaches won't get an aura and tension headaches don't tend to inflame the blood vessels.

2) Treatments for Tension Headaches

How to treat Tension Headaches

Tension headache treatment often concentrates on pain relieving medication. There are several medications that are prescribed for patients suffering from chronic tension type headaches. There are also some over-the-counter medications that can be used. Some of the medications that are suggested for the treatment of tension type headaches are detailed in the next section.

There are many drugs that can be prescribed when it comes to tension headache medication, so if the medication you are currently prescribed isn't working, talk to your doctor about alternatives, and don't feel as though you are limited to one form of treatment.

The type of tension headaches treatment that you are prescribed will depend on a lot of individual factors. Here are some of the most common types of medication for tension headaches along with their possible side effects.

3) Tension Headaches - Medication

a) Fioricet

Fioricet is one of the drugs that is often prescribed for the symptoms of tension headaches; many patients find this drug effective. As well as containing a barbiturate, it also contains acetaminophen, which acts to reduce pain. In addition, caffeine is included as an added ingredient.

Side Effects:

Some patients report becoming too dependent on this drug due to a barbiturate called butalbital contained in it.

b) Tricyclic Medications

Tricyclic medications are used most often to treat depression. However, these medications are also helpful in reducing some types of pain and are sometimes prescribed for the treatment of tension headaches. Tricyclic medications come in various forms; some of the most common ones are amitriptyline and nortriptyline. Doctors often advise that these medications are taken at night as they will also act to help improve sleep and taking this medication at night-time is useful for patients who tend to wake up with a tension-type headache or patients who experience discomfort during the night.

Side Effects:

This type of medication can cause side effects such as a dry mouth, upset stomach or dizziness. Some patients also report an increase in appetite. There might also be other side effects associated with this drug, but not all patients will be affected by them.

Some patients on this type of medication might find that they have a sedative effect, and for that reason it is advised that patients don't drive after taking them or operate heavy machinery.

Patients might also experience some uncomfortable side effects such as dizziness when coming off this drug. If your doctor decides that you no longer need this kind of medication, then they will advise you to come off it slowly in order to minimise the withdrawal symptoms.

These types of medications aren't usually prescribed to patients who are on levothyroxine as they can interact with thyroid medication.

c) Nurofen Tension Headache

Several brands now produce medication specifically as a treatment for tension headache. Nurofen Tension Headache Relief is just one of a number of over-the-counter treatments for tension headaches. The medication is a combination of Ibuprofen and lysine and can be helpful for trying to manage the pain yourself.

However, patients with an underlying medical condition should consult their doctor before buying any over-the-counter medication in case there are any contraindications with the medications they are already on.

Side Effects:

It is advisable not to take anti-inflammatory medications or NSAIDS long term as they can cause stomach problems. They can also cause problems with bleeding so, for this reason, they might not be prescribed to patients on blood thinning medication. Other side effects reported while using this type of medication include sickness and nausea

Another over-the-counter medication is Excedrin for tension headaches. The medication also works to relieve neck and shoulder pain and has the active ingredient acetaminophen; it also includes added caffeine. Excedrin for migraine sufferers is also available.

d) Melatonin

Melatonin is a hormone that is produced by the pineal gland as we sleep. However, in some people this hormone is depleted and some headache sufferers have been found to be low in melatonin, which is why it is believed that melatonin can be effective in relieving tension headaches in some patients.

Melatonin is often prescribed for patients suffering from insomnia but it has also been found to be beneficial in treating tension headaches and migraines.

Side Effects:

Some patients taking melatonin experience various aches and pains and inflammations. Some patients also have stomach pain while taking this medication and some will have periods of insomnia and dizziness.

There are more serious side effects to taking melatonin and if any patient has side effects that are too severe, then they should talk to their medical team.

4) What Causes Tension Headaches?

The causes of tension headaches can be many and varied. Tension type headaches are often caused by stress. However, they can also be down to a number of other factors, which are detailed in this next section. Tension type headaches can also be down to lifestyle and posture so these are issues that will all need to be addressed if the patient is to see an improvement in their symptoms or at least lessen the number of headaches that they have. There are also a number of other factors that can contribute to tension headaches that are detailed below and if a patient is experiencing daily tension headaches they should ensure that they address all of the following factors.

If you want to understand how to ease tension headaches, then you need to understand the factors that can contribute to them. Listed below are some of the common tension headache causes.

a) Stress

Stress can often be a major cause of tension headaches. These headaches might occur while the person is stressed or after they have suffered a stressful period in their life. Most people will have different ways of unwinding and reducing stress such as listening to music, practicing yoga or spending time with friends and (or "or") family.

If you know that there is going to be a stressful time ahead at work or at home, then make sure you work some time into your schedule to properly manage the stress. Use any of the above options as a way of relaxing or find something else that you enjoy doing.

Meditation and Cognitive Behavioural Therapy, or CBT, are popular ways of helping the mind and body to cope with stress. Meditation will help the person to feel more focused and better able to cope with their workload.

b) Sleep

The power of a good night's sleep cannot be underestimated. Most people will be familiar with the groggy feeling that they experience when they haven't had enough sleep and this feeling of being under par will continue throughout the day.

When a person suffers from a lack of sleep, not only will this lead to aches and pains all over, but it will mean that the body will release a hormone called cortisol to help the body cope with the effects of stress. If someone lacks a good night's rest over a long period of time then this can lead to them being under constant stress and leave them more vulnerable to headaches.

Make sure that you have a proper routine at bedtime, perhaps try a few gentle stretches to release the neck and shoulder area before sleep and try using a meditation or creative visualisation CD last thing at night to wind down and get the body ready for a restful sleep.

c) Eyestrain

Eyestrain is another major cause of tension headaches. If you notice that the tension headaches are occurring after long periods in front of the computer then make sure that you are taking regular breaks. If your eyes feel tired when you are working then this is one of the major symptoms of eyestrain and it is a sign that you really need to take a break.

To reduce the chance of eyestrain, don't go for more than 15-20 minutes without taking a break. Make sure that the room or office that you are working from is well lit and don't work until the point that you are overtired and can't see clearly what you are writing.

If the symptoms of eyestrain continue, make an appointment with an optician. They can prescribe lenses that are suitable for close work and they might suggest tinted lenses to reduce (or "minimise") the glare from the screen.

d) Neck and Shoulder Tension

Carrying excess tension in the neck and shoulders will inevitably lead to the development of headaches. Make sure when you are using a computer that your shoulders aren't being hunched up and take regular breaks to stretch out the neck and shoulder muscles.

Simple exercises such as gently turning the neck from side to side will help reduce neck pain or swinging the arms from side to side will help to relax tension that has gathered in the shoulder area.

If excess shoulder tension is a problem for you then perhaps see a massage therapist as they will be able to concentrate on these areas of tension and help to reduce any muscle spasm that might have occurred in the neck or shoulders.

e) Computer Work

Spending long hours in front of a computer, whether it is for leisure or work purposes, will often cause tension headaches to occur. Sitting in one position for any length of time will lead to tension accumulating in the shoulders and the neck, thus contributing to the development of a headache.

The sitting position while at a computer can also cause tension type headaches to develop. Make sure that you don't sit slumped at your desk and sit with your spine straight; a back cushion or an ergonomic chair will help with this.

In addition, make sure that the monitor is at eye level so that you don't have to stare down at the screen as this will cause pain in the neck and upper back area.

f) Posture

Posture is another contributor to tension headaches. People get used to holding themselves in a certain way and they often don't notice the areas of tension that they are carrying around with them. Make sure that you walk tall, stand and sit straight and sit with the feet flat on the floor to avoid tension building in the lower back.

Take time out to check that your shoulders aren't hunched as this can become the natural position for some people, often without them even noticing. Roll your shoulders several times a day to stop tension building in this area.

In addition, check the position of your neck when you walk, or ask a friend to check for you. Sometimes, the neck can be tilted slightly to the side when a person walks. This is sometimes a sign of a neck spasm and, although pain might not have started at this point, it soon will. A massage therapist will be able to address this type of problem.

g) Jaw Problems

If you often wake up in the morning with a tense feeling in the back of the head and pain around the jaw and face, then this is a sure sign that you are clenching or grinding your teeth at night. This often happens when a person is stressed or anxious about something, but it can also be a sign of excess tension.

Problems with the jaw or teeth might not be one of the most obvious causes of severe headaches, but this is something that should be explored if a patient hasn't found anything else that could be causing their pain.

Check your teeth, especially the lower ones. If they look slightly worn down, then you are clenching your teeth at night and if they are ground down, then you are grinding the teeth at night, and this will cause pain throughout the jaw and head area.

Fortunately, this can be remedied by wearing a mouth guard at night and learning to manage stress and anxiety. If the problems continue, your dentist might refer you to a jaw specialist. During an appointment with a specialist, they will check to see how well the jaw is working and look for any problem areas.

Some patients will be referred on to a physiotherapist to get exercises to help restore the normal function of the jaw or it will be suggested that they try massage therapy to help reduce any spasms in the jaw, head or neck area.

h) Tension Headaches and Alcohol

While many people find drinking alcohol to be relaxing, alcohol is known to be associated with tension headaches, so this should be drunk in moderation if you find that it makes the pain worse or causes more tension headaches.

In addition, if a patient is already taking medication for headaches, then they should be aware that some medications can make the effects of alcohol stronger, which could, in turn, make a headache worse.

i) Smoking

Smoking is another bad habit that you might want to curb if you suffer from tension type headaches. Some people like to relax with a cigarette, especially when they are stressed. However, it is much better to look at ways to deal with stress naturally.

j) Caffeine

Everyone reacts to caffeine differently, and while some people can tolerate a seemingly endless amount of caffeine without any problems, some people find that drinking caffeinated drinks will cause headaches.

Others find that coming off caffeine will also lead to the development of tension type headaches. The problem with caffeine is although it does have some health benefits, if you are already stressed, then consuming extra caffeine will make the mind feel even more anxious and irritated.

5) Tension - Symptoms

Perhaps one of the most effective ways of managing these types of headaches is to be aware of the first signs of tension. Muscle tension and headache go hand in hand, so preventing the muscles from becoming tight and tense is vital for reducing the number of tension headaches.

People can often detect tension just by looking at how they hold themselves. One of the first places for tension to accumulate is in the shoulders, so make sure that your shoulders aren't hunched and make sure that your arms swing freely and that the movement in your neck isn't limited.

Tension will nearly always be felt as pain so if you have pain in the neck or shoulder area, then you are holding tension there.

Chapter 11) Home Remedies for Tension Type Headaches

Although the causes of a tension headache will often vary from person to person, there are several factors that often lead to the development of tension headaches and there are a number of steps that people can take that have been found to be effective. In this chapter, you'll find several effective home remedies for headaches and find tips on how to relieve a tension headache.

1) Water

Drinking plain water could be the most basic tension headache home remedy. Dehydration can help contribute to a tension type headache. Although consuming extra water might not work for everyone, some people notice a reduction in headaches when they increase their water intake.

The experts say that we should be drinking 6-8 glasses of water every day. This is especially important for people who work in front of computers all day, people who work or live in stuffy or humid environments and people who undertake a lot of activity.

Consuming that much water every day can seem like a bit of a challenge, but by drinking a glass of water at break times, and taking a bottle of water to drink at lunchtime or throughout the day, it is much easier.

For people who don't like the taste of tap water, a water filter jug is ideal. Once the jug is filled with fresh water, leave it to sit in the fridge for a bit while the chlorine taste that is sometimes present fades away.

2) Caffeine

It might not seem like the obvious solution, but caffeine has been shown to reduce tension headaches in some people. Caffeine has also been shown to be more effective when taken alongside Ibuprofen. Ibuprofen is often sold in combination with caffeine as it helps the drug to act faster and provide better pain relief. However, some headaches sufferers find that caffeine can increase the incidences of headache, and suddenly withdrawing caffeine from the diet can also have the same effect.

In addition, many people find that caffeine makes them hyper, and this can lead to anxiety and tension.

3) Fresh air

A stuffy environment can often cause tension headaches and many people develop a headache when the atmosphere is close. If you are at home, try and keep the windows open where you can and keep the interior doors open as well so that there is a fresh flow of air running through the house.
If you feel a tension headache beginning to develop, go outdoors into the fresh air and see if the change of environment makes a difference. A walk in the fresh air will also allow any stress to dissipate and is one of the easiest tension headache remedies to work into your schedule.

4) Self-Massage

Self-massage techniques are perfect for reducing the tension in the neck or head area and are helpful when the first signs of a tension headache begin to appear. This form of massage can be carried out anytime or any place and should be done when the first signs of tension start to show. Self-massage can also be used to provide relief for a tension headache once it has begun.

To do a self-massage, use the knuckles to carefully massage the temples and any other areas of tension across the forehead. This can be done with massage oils, but it can also be done without them or with a rubbing balm.

To massage the neck, place both hands in the back of the neck, and make small circular motions with the fingers.

5) Aspirin

Aspirin has been found to be an effective way of treating tension type headaches and it is an inexpensive tension headache remedy, so make sure that there's always some available for when you need it.

Medications like aspirin should not be taken to excess as it can cause stomach bleeding, so don't depend on this form of medication too often. Moreover, when taken for a long time, over- the-counter medications such as aspirin can cause headaches.

6) Ice Packs

Placing an ice pack on the tense muscles that cause a tension headache can be an effective remedy for a tension headache. Whether the tension is in the temples, the neck or the shoulders, an ice pack can help to alleviate the discomfort and relax the muscles.

Ice packs that have been designed for sports injuries are readily available and these are compact enough to place on tight tense muscles and they can help provide relief from tension headaches.

7) Heat packs

Some people cannot tolerate ice and find that the action of placing ice on a tense muscle can cause the muscle to tense further still, causing more pain.

If this is the case, then a heat pack is the best alternative to relieve tension headaches and it will allow the tight muscles to relax, relieving the tense feeling that will ultimately lead to a tension headache if it is left untreated.

8) Rubbing Balms

These balms come in compact tins and are perfect for keeping with you throughout the day and they can be effective in the treatment of a tension headache. They are small enough to fit into a pocket and they are a convenient way of treating the early stages of a tension headache; these are also available in stick form.

There are various different balms available, however, the mind balm for stress or the night balm are the best options. These products are completely natural and have essential oils that are known to have a relaxing affect.

Rub a little bit of the balm into the temples, the nape of the neck or any area of the head where tension is accumulating.

Alternatively, people can make their own balms for a unique, soothing balm with the essential oils of their choice. Instructions on how to do this are included at the back of the book.

9) Calming the Breath

Calming the breath can help to ease stress and tension naturally and can be one of the most natural cures for headaches. Taking a few minutes to steady the breath will slow it down and allow the mind to calm, helping to ease any stressful thoughts that might be occurring.

Slow, steady breathing will also slow the heart rate and help to lower the blood pressure, which will usually rise when a person is stressed. Learning to calm the breath will also help to reduce the surge in cortisol that occurs when a person is feeling stressed and panicked.

A useful way to become more aware of the way that you breathe is meditation. Many CDs teach breath counting as a form of meditation and this is something that, once learned properly, can be used whenever it is needed.

10) Kava Balm

This balm can be beneficial to patients when they experience the first signs and symptoms of tension headaches as the massage effect of the balm will also help to relax the muscles.

This balm has a relaxing effect and is best used last thing at night. It has rather a strong scent, which some people might not like, but it does help to aid a relaxing night's sleep.

Some people also experience strange dreams while using Kava. It should not be used by people taken medication for mental illness. If you are unsure whether Kava is suitable for you, then speak to your doctor first.

Chapter 12) Alternative Therapies for Tension Headaches

Alternative therapies can be helpful in reducing the stress that often leads to tension headaches. These therapies are considered safe enough to be used regularly and they will have a relaxing effect on the entire body. Many of the therapies will have a calming effect on the mind too, helping to counter stress and reduce the occurrence of tension headaches.

The following options offer a natural approach to the treatment of a tension headache.

1) Aromatherapy

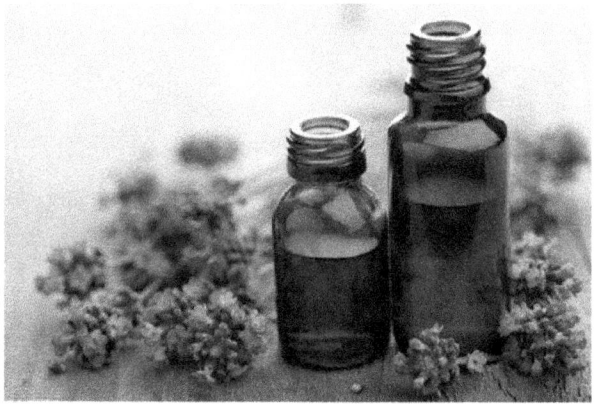

Aromatherapy is an affordable way to help alleviate the symptoms of a tension headache. While some of the essential oils can be a little bit pricey, they last an extremely long time, so it is worth the once off purchase.

Essential oils are good for using last thing at night as part of a relaxation routine. The oils can be stored in a screw top jar and they will keep for several weeks.

To get the most out of the oils, make sure that there is a high concentration of the active ingredient so that you can gain more benefit from the effects. Don't buy inexpensive oils, as these sometimes don't have much of the active ingredient in them, and buy well-known brands.

Some of the contraindications for each oil are also detailed. However, before using any of the oils, it is best to speak to your doctor first in case you are on medication or have a health condition that could be affected by the use of these oils. Pregnant and breast feeding women should also take advice before using any of the oils.

There are several essential oils that are beneficial for people suffering from tension headaches. Detailed below are some of the essential oils that are often used to aid relaxation and reduce tension.

a) Lavender
Lavender can be used by adding a few drops to some base oil, by putting a few drops in while the bath is running, or by adding a few drops on the pillow.

It can also be used in ready-mixed solutions and usually comes with a blend of other oils that are known to assist the relaxation process. When it is mixed with base oil, lavender is safe to massage onto the skin.

When using lavender essential oil as part of a massage, concentrate on the temples, which can often gather tension and on the back of the neck. The shoulders should also be massaged too.

Contraindications:

Pregnant and nursing women should not use this oil. It should not be used by patients on cholesterol lowering or blood thinning medication and patients on anti-depressant and anti-convulsant drugs, or on any form of sedatives, should not use this oil.

b) Chamomile

Chamomile is a well-known sleep aid and can be bought individually or as part of a combination of oils. The oil can be used in much the same way as the lavender oil and can be added to the bath, dropped onto the pillow or added to a base oil.

Again, concentrate on areas of the upper body that gather tension. This will often be different for everyone, but the main areas to focus on will be the temples, neck and shoulders.

Contraindications:

Patients with an underlying medical condition, pregnant women or patients on any form of medication should seek advice before using the oil.

c) Ylang Ylang

Ylang Ylang is a beautifully scented, uplifting essential oil. It has mood lifting properties and it can help to reduce feelings of stress and anxiety. However, aroma therapist Linda Southall warns that this oil does have a strong aroma and can cause headaches and nausea in some people, especially when used in large concentrations.

To use the oil, use it sparingly, and add some Ylang Ylang essential oils to some base oil then massage into the skin.

d) Peppermint

The refreshing aroma of peppermint essential oil will help to clear a headache and it is good for congestion, too.

Contraindications:

Linda Southall advises people to use in low concentrations as it may irritate sensitive skin. It is not to be used if there is a history of heart disease or epilepsy. Do not use this oil if pregnant or taking homeopathic remedies.

e) Basil

Basil works well to help ease stress-related headaches and it can be an effective treatment for a headache. The oil can be blended with lemongrass.

Contraindications:

The oil should not be used by pregnant women, patients who suffer from epilepsy/seizures or by people with high blood pressure.

f) Rosemary

Rosemary essential oil has a refreshing fragrance that can be useful to help clear headaches.

Contraindications:

Rosemary is not to be used by people who may be pregnant, have high blood pressure or epilepsy.

g) Melissa

Melissa essential oil is known for its refreshing lemony scent. It is also known as lemon balm.

Melissa is especially helpful for migraine and stress headaches. It is an effective anti-spasmodic and nerve tonic. The oil is also known to aid sleep and ease restlessness; however, it is very expensive oil.

h) Eucalyptus

This oil has quite a strong fragrance and it is especially useful for headaches that have developed following a cold or sinus infection.

Adding a few drops to some hot water and inhaling the vapour is useful for relieving congestion in the head and it will help to relieve blocked sinuses.

Contraindications:

The oil shouldn't be used by pregnant women, people with high blood pressure or epilepsy. The oil is also too strong to be used by young children and it is advisable to not use the oil before surgery.

i) Mixed Blends

If you don't want to mix your own oils, then mixed blends make effective headache treatments. These often come in stick or roller ball form and can be used throughout the day, whenever you can feel tension building.

Applying these also has a cooling, calming effect and the small containers that the mixed blends come in means that they are idea for carrying around in a handbag or pocket.

These can be applied to the wrists and other pulse points whenever you feel the need.

Oils such as peppermint and rosemary are also good for reducing tension headaches. They can be massaged into the hairline and into the shoulders, but don't use them neat on the skin.

2) Osteopathy

Osteopathy has proven to be an effective way of treating headaches and managing the shoulder and neck problems that contribute to them. Tim Allardyce, MCSP SRP, is an Osteopath at Croydon Physio. He explains what to expect when you visit an osteopath for treatment for the first time and how an osteopath can help in the treatment of headache and the related symptoms.

"An osteopath will look at your body in a holistic way, to work out the cause of your pain. Osteopaths believe that everything in the body is there for a reason, and is underpinned by three philosophies: 1) Structure governs function (meaning that the structure of the body is there for a purpose, for a function). 2) The rule of the artery is supreme – if we normalise blood flow in the body, we will stimulate healing as blood delivers oxygen and metabolites necessary for cell repair. 3) The body produces its own medicines, and is capable of self-healing if given the right conditions.

 "During your first treatment we will take a case history. This involves asking you questions about how your injury/pain occurred, when it occurred, which things make it worse, and which things make it better. We will also ask you about sports, work and hobbies that you do that might affect your condition. We will also ask about your previous medical history, such as serious illnesses, or previous similar problems. After this, we will do a physical examination. This includes looking at your muscles and bone structure, posture, and checking your range of movement. We might ask you to bend, side-bend, or rotate to check how mobile your joints are. We will also palpate your muscles to determine how tight they are.

"Once the examination is complete, we will discuss with you what the diagnosis is, and how the condition is most effectively treated. Assuming that no further tests or examinations are required, treatment will then commence, and usually involves manual hands-on therapy."

Tim also explains how osteopathy is used to treat headaches.

"The first question that needs to be asked by your osteopath is: "What is causing the headaches?" It could be that a certain food allergy, stress or psychological illness, hormones, posture, or muscle tension is the causative factor. If your osteopath feels that the neck, posture, or muscle tension is the cause, they will treat the relevant area to relieve your headaches. A significant number of headaches can be attributed to the neck. When neck muscles get tight, it can restrict blood flow to the head, and also pinch on nerves going to the head causing the pain of headaches. There is a particularly naughty group of muscles that sit just below the back of the skull called the suboccipital muscles. This group of four small muscles can get very tight, causing referred pain into the back of the head and then over to the eyes and frontal part of the head.

"We are also seeing an increased prevalence of office workers suffering headaches, especially those who spend long hours with their neck bent forwards. Computer monitors are a big problem too, when they are too low it places the neck in a poor postural position, placing strain on the neck muscles and ligaments. Laptop use is the other big cause, encouraging people to bend their neck forwards. Another common cause is stress, as the muscles in the neck tighten when we are tense, especially when hunching our shoulders.

"So how do we treat your headaches?

"We have many techniques in our tool box to use to relieve your headaches. The most common is massage to release muscle tension in the head and neck. The second is joint mobilisation. When the neck is stiff, you are more likely to suffer headaches, so improving range of mobility to your neck using manual techniques can reduce your headaches. Sometimes we use traction, to stretch the neck, and relieve pressure on the joints, discs, and muscles. We will also look at ways of improving your posture. Typically people with bad posture will more likely suffer headaches as the neck is put into a mechanically poor position. This is known as forward head posture, and puts the neck under enormous strain. By correcting posture with soft tissue techniques and exercises, we can relieve the strain on your head. Other tools sometimes used include acupuncture, and ultrasound.

"But that is not all we will do:

"Being holistic practitioners, we will look to discuss ways to improve your lifestyle. So we might need you to change your workstation set up, or cut out certain foods in your diet, or do exercises to strengthen your neck, or give you strategies to reduce stress. All of these combined with treatment to your neck can make a super powerful natural headache cure. I cure about 90% of headaches using these techniques, so you can see that it's very successful as a form of treatment, and also very safe without the need for medication."

6 top tips to fix headaches:

- Use a laptop stand – for less than £30 you can raise your laptop and it puts less strain through the neck.
- Raise your monitor by 4 inches – it will help keep you upright, and stop your neck bending forwards so much.
- Use a document holder to stop repetitive forward neck bending and extending. Keeping your documents at eye level will reduce the constant bending and extending.
- Hold your iPad and iPhone up high when using them for long periods.
- Reduce stress – suboccipital muscles are affected by stress, so reducing stress can reduce the tension in these muscles. Learn to relax your shoulders to reduce the tension in the neck muscles.
- See an osteopath or physiotherapist; many have experience treating headaches.

3) Chinese Medicine

Acupuncture for tension headaches is an approach that is commonly used in Chinese medicine. Here, the theory behind Chinese medicine is explained.

a) A Key Concept in the Theoretical Background of Chinese Medicine – Brief Outline

The basic principle of Chinese Medical treatment is that a living human body contains vital energy (Qi) which circulates inside via discreet pathways. When these flows of energy are blocked or unbalanced, pain and illness arise. This vital energy is partly inherited from parents but must also be acquired from food and oxygen. The acquired Qi can be viewed as the essential nutrient carried by the bloodstream across the body. Given their interlinked roles, blood and Qi should be viewed collectively and in Chinese Medicine the latter is known as 'the shadow' of the former. Therefore a concept of 'lifeblood' can be helpful in understanding the Chinese Medical view that a constant circulation of energy is crucial to sustaining good health.

b) Tension Headaches – Diagnosis and Treatment

Chinese Medicine offers various methods of providing cures for tension headaches.

In Chinese Medical terms, tension headache would be recognised as an empty type of headache produced by an internal cause. There are several syndromes where tension headache would arise as a symptom: Stomach- and Spleen-Qi Deficiency, Kidney Deficiency (shortage of essential energy within the Kidneys); accumulation of Dampness or Stomach Heat (excess heat within the stomach).

According to the syndrome identified at the root of patient's tension headaches, acupuncture points and Chinese herbs would be used to replenish the essential energy within the stomach, spleen and kidneys; or eliminate the excess dampness or heat from the body.

4) Homeopathic Remedies for Headaches

Homeopathy isn't for everyone but many patients believe that it works for them. There are several homeopathic remedies that are suggested for tension-type headaches, and migraines. However, as everyone will have different symptoms, and the headaches will vary in intensity, it is best to go and see a homeopath who can suggest a suitable remedy for your particular symptoms.

5) Massage Therapy

Massage is a useful tool to relieve tension headaches. People who suffer from these types of headaches can try some self-massage techniques as described in the home remedies for tension headaches chapter. However, if you suffer from chronic tension in the neck and shoulder area then a regular session with a physiotherapist or massage therapist will be useful for helping to reduce tightness and spasms in the neck and shoulder area.

Patients can self-refer to a massage therapist or to a physiotherapist in their local area. They can often see patients within 24-48 hours, which is helpful to those patients with frequent tension headaches.

6) Chiropractor

A chiropractor can help to address any issues involving posture that might be contributing to tension-type headaches. If headache and tension has become an on-going issue, then a chiropractor will be able to help establish if there are any underlying postural issues that are triggering the tension headaches.

Chapter 13) Herbs for Relaxation

As reducing tension and stress can help aid sufferers of tension type headaches, this chapter will detail some of the herbs that can be used for reducing stress and the build-up of tension. Some of these herbs are also useful for treating headaches.

As the herbs detailed have a sedative effect, and as they can sometimes have side effects, they should not be taken if you are already on any prescribed medications. It is imperative to get medical advice first as your doctor is best placed to ascertain if these herbal remedies for headaches/stress relief are a suitable approach for you.

Moreover, due to the sedative effects of the herbs listed, it is advisable not to use them if you are going to drive or if you will be operating heavy machinery.

1) Passionflower

Passionflower helps to relieve tension and stress. The herb can also help to ease anxiety and calm the mind so that it is easier to relax. The calming effect that passionflower has on the mind slows down the rate of thoughts, especially if someone has repetitive, stressful thoughts: for example, a problem that they keep mulling over, which makes it difficult to quieten the mind.

Passionflower can be taken as a tea and the soothing aroma will also help to calm the emotions. Try inhaling the aroma to reduce any feelings of tension in the head. Passionflower can also be taken in tablet form. They can be taken throughout the day and last thing at night to help ease the mind and calm agitation before bedtime.

These herbal tablets are non-addictive and ideal for people who want to soothe their mind without depending too much on medication.

The herb can also be brought as a tincture, as drops, or as combination with other relaxing herbs.

2) St John's Wort

St John's Wort has long been used as a herbal remedy for minor depression. As well as lifting moods, the herb can help to ease anxiety and tension.

It can be brought in the form of tablets, capsules, a tincture or a tea.

The herb shouldn't be taken by people who are already on anti-depressant medication or by women who are using contraceptives. Pregnant and breast feeding women should also take advice before supplementing their diet with this herb.

3) Lemon Balm

Lemon balm is a herb that is well-known for its soothing, relaxing effects and it is commonly used to help ease stress and anxiety; it is also useful for aiding a restful sleep. It can help soothe the mind, lift the mood and help to relieve tension and it is one of the popular remedies for tension headaches.

Due to the calming effect that lemon balm has on the mind, it is ideal for drinking as a tea during the day or late evening/ last thing at night to aid relaxation before bedtime.

Lemon balm can be bought as a tea or bought as capsules. It is also available as part of a combination mixed with other relaxing herbs. It's a useful herb to take throughout the day in low doses to help combat stress.

The tea can be drunk hot or cold. To drink the tea cold, prepare as usual, allow to cool, then put it in the fridge and serve with ice cubes when you are ready to drink it. Don't add the ice cubes if you are prone to sinus headaches.

4) Green Tea

The soothing, calming properties of green tea will help the mind to become more relaxed. The tea is also full of antioxidants and it is believed to have many other health benefits, such as helping diabetics to lower their blood sugar.

There is a caffeine free version for those who find caffeine either triggers a headache or makes them feel jittery and stressed. There are also many flavoured versions of teas to choose from if you don't like the taste of green tea.

5) Jasmine

Jasmine can be brought in combination with green tea and has an uplifting, calming effect on the mind. This tea is extremely effective at helping to lift the mood and it will help to ease anxiety.

6) Chamomile

Chamomile has been used for centuries for the calming effect it can have on the mind and body. The aromatic scent of this tea is enough to start gently calming the mind and drinking the tea at times of stress or anxiety can help the mind to calm, which will then make it easier to think about a stressful situation much more rationally.

Chamomile is the ideal tea for drinking early evening or last thing at night to help aid sleep. Some people don't like the taste of chamomile as it can take a bit of getting used to. However, it can be bought with flavours such as spearmint or it can be bought as a night-time tea that also contains a mix of other calming herbs.

7) Hops

Hops are usually used to flavour beer, but they have medicinal properties too. Hops are a popular remedy for people who suffer from anxiety, which makes them a valuable relaxation aid. Hops can also be used to aid sleep and they are useful for when people are feeling unsettled or nervous.

Hops can be brought as part of a combination of herbs, usually in products that are designed to promote sleep naturally, or hops can be used as a hop pillow and placed under the usual pillow to help aid sleep.

Using hops in this way can help alleviate anxiety and will reduce the chances of a person grinding or clenching their teeth at night, which can help prevent tension-type headaches.

Some people can have an allergic reaction to hops and can often get a small red rash after taking them, so be mindful of this before using.

8) Valerian

Valerian has long been used as a powerful relaxant and the herb has been used for centuries to help promote relaxation. As well as being used to help promote a relaxed sleep, valerian can help to reduce anxiety and agitation.

The herb can be brought as standardised capsules, a tincture or as a tea. It can also be brought in a combination with other herbs for relaxation. Night-time tea mixtures often contain valerian as well.

There can be some side effects with valerian with some people reporting stomach ache or a feeling of depression after consuming it.

Chapter 14) Self-hypnosis, NLP and Stress

Marilyn Devonish is a Certified Master Practitioner and Trainer of Neuro Linguistic Programming (NLP), Certified Trainer of Hypnosis, Certified Trainer of Time Line Therapy, Certified PhotoReading and Accelerated Learning, and a Practitioner of various other modalities including EFT, Huna, Positive EFT, Energetic NLP, DNA Theta Healing, EmoTrance, Soul Planning, and Archetypal Profiling.

In this chapter, Marilyn Devonish explains some useful techniques for combating stress.

Stress in its purest form is almost the body being out of equilibrium and balance or being pushed beyond the limit of what the system feels it was designed to do. From the neurological perspective the sympathetic nervous system, the body's 'fight or flight' response is over stimulated, and is characterised by physical factors such as increased heart rate, constricted blood vessels and a rush of adrenalin. In psychological terms it can be characterised by emotions such as fear, anxiety, frustration, and anger.

Because of the arousal of the sympathetic nervous system, one of the first things that I would recommend when working with clients who don't respond well in stressful situations is to activate the parasympathetic nervous system, which is the body's natural relaxation response. The parasympathetic nervous system slows the heart rate, dilates the blood vessels, and allows for an increase in blood flow. This simple yet powerful exercise is a blend of what I teach my PhotoReading™ students, or running Presentation Skills Classes, both of which are environments that people tend to find highly stressful.

1. Take a deep breath in and exhale, and repeat this half a dozen or so times. This increases the oxygen flow around the body as well as sending a good supply of oxygen to stimulate the brain and help you think more clearly.

2. Get into peripheral vision or expanded awareness. When the body is under stress people automatically go into tunnel vision which starts to close down their awareness and focus in on the stressful situation and uses the more analytical part of the brain. Although great for those life threatening decisions, it is not so great for coming up with creative ideas or solutions because the right side of the brain takes a bit of a back seat. Being in expanded awareness encourages left and right brain integration and enables clearer thinking and increases the likelihood of being able to come up with ideas or a solution. To check whether you are in peripheral vision, find a point to look at straight ahead, and whilst continuing to look straight ahead put your hands at either side of you head (much like you used to do as a child if you were going to stick your tongue out at someone) and then wiggle your fingers. If you can see your fingers moving without turning your head you are in peripheral vision. For those that are more into esoteric studies, in Hawaiian Huna terms, this is also referred to as the state of Hakalau, and is one of the Huna meditative practices.

3. Imagine a point located about 6 inches above and slightly behind the head and focus on that for a few moments. This helps to harness random thoughts and focus the mind. (This step is also a great process for those suffering with dyslexia, which in itself can be very stressful, particularly when people are attempting to keep it a secret).

As I noted earlier this relates to people who don't respond well in stressful situations. Stress and anxiety are also determined by our response to it, and the meaning that we assign. Some people often mistakenly see the stress as a source of fuel or internal motivation. This might be true in the short term, if however they don't have the capacity to deal with it, things can get out of control and it becomes a hindrance rather than a help.

1) NLP

There are several techniques from the field of NLP which are designed to help deal with stress and anxiety. A few of these include:

a) Changing the Internal Representation or Submodality

For example when I used to be terrified of spiders, and public speaking, the internal picture immediately invoked high levels of fear and stress. The picture in my mind was super large, I was seeing every awful moment and movement of those multiple legs through my own eyes, it was almost dark and muted with lots of lurking shadows, and there was a heaviness to it in the pit of the stomach, and a wave of panic that extended from the stomach through to the heart. An NLP Trainer or Practitioner would work with changing what are known as the Submodalies of the internal representation so that it no longer invokes an internal stress response, and mapping the old feelings across to the new state. The premise is that you think about the characteristics of something that you enjoy or find relaxing. The internal representation for the things that you enjoy will have key factors, which are vastly different to the first scenario.

b) Anchoring Resourceful State

A popular methodology can be to anchor positive or resourceful states. The anchor can be a movement, a gesture, even a word which has associated to it how you want to respond instead. For example, in some sporting activities the competitors always enter the arena to a particular piece of music, which is an example of an anchor, something which invokes a state more conducive to the task in hand. Other people might have their lucky mascot or a gesture like punching the air and shouting 'yessss!'

c) Limiting Beliefs

There can often be deeper underlying causes of stress and anxiety. Common beliefs that I encounter which limit a persons' ability to deal with a stressful situation, include not being, or should I say not feeling, good enough, clever enough, capable enough, worthy enough. These beliefs act as a filter through which people see the world and judge their performance or ability to perform in certain areas. For example, when I held the belief that I wasn't good enough, my anxiety around public speaking was heightened because I began to question why anyone would even be remotely interested in what I had to say, and even if they were, I believed that I would more than likely have made a fool of myself. Unearthing and resolving these unhelpful beliefs gives a whole new perspective on your ability to achieve things from a place of relaxation, ease and flow.

Identify the root cause. Aside from an array of techniques, of which there are hundreds I could choose from, one of the key things that I am interested in when working with a client is the root cause of the condition. From a therapeutic point of view, it might also be referred to as 'secondary gain', meaning an underlying benefit of having things be this way. People will often initially object and can give 101 reasons why what they are experiencing is a problem and has no positive benefit or gain whatsoever. When you can identify the root cause of an issue and find a more ecological and healthy way to satisfy those needs, the stress response can disappear. For example, I had a client who used to get the most terrible migraine headaches which of course seemed purely physical. The underlying secondary gain, however, was that the migraine meant they had to take some time out and have a rest, something which under normal circumstances they would rarely give themselves permission to do.

When we started identifying additional ways in which to take time out, the migraines also started to disappear. The same is true for something like public speaking. The secondary gain might be to stop you from making a fool of yourself, so the mind and body will invoke a response to save you from this terrible fate. The resulting sabotage of course contributes to you falling into the very trap that you want to avoid, however that is not the first concern of the inner mind, whose primary function is to save you from the underlying apparent threat.

2) Reframing and Hypnosis

A little like working with the internal representation and Submodalities, although less process driven, is changing the frame of reference and having the stress triggers mean something else. Part of it is about changing your point of view. For example, when you change and link the thought of standing on stage in front of 1,000 people to something that is associated to relaxation and fun, and a way of helping people by imparting important information, everything changes.

a) A Few Simple Questions

I have found that it is also vital to really identify what sits beneath the stress and what the mind and body are attempting to get people to pay attention to. The following questions are very powerful ways to start looking at that:

- What is it that you need to know, learn or pay attention to?
- When you learn and pay attention to it, can you resolve it now?

- What is the stress or anxiety trying to get for you or allow you to do?

Go with whatever responses come to mind and keep going. The real gems tend to show up after you hit what I call the void. To really externalise it, say it out loud or write it down.

Are you creating drama or trauma? Also pay attention to the stories that you create around these situations. People often add to a small issue and build a ton of drama around it, such that it almost becomes part of their psyche and identity. Take a moment to consider:

- Who would you be without the drama?
- What will you do if the drama and story were to now disappear?

This can be most enlightening and often reveals to people that they fear they will lose part of their identity without it because they have become so used to it. For some, much as it is causing them real problems, they almost wouldn't have anything to talk about or focus on anymore.

b) Identify the Opposite
The mind often doesn't like a void so if you try to remove the anxiety but there is nothing to replace it people often find that the problem will eventually return. I always ask my clients: If you didn't have anxiety or stress (insert your own stuff here) what would you choose to have instead? The first response that I usually get is a list of what they don't want: They wouldn't be stressed, nervous, anxious, fearful, scared, sick, etc. What you want to do is identify what you actually do want; this might include feeling more relaxed, confident, engaged, etc. This not only shifts the internal representation and focus, it also has a big neurological impact and will start to create the corresponding

feelings. (Try it: If you have any kind of fear or phobia, spiders, pigeons, heights etc., and notice how quickly the mere thought affects your neurology and invokes a stress response).

In a nutshell relax the body, expand your awareness, ask what you need to be aware of or pay attention to, and resolve any underlying fears or anxieties. This then creates the capacity to choose and decide your next move and response.

People often ask how long it actually takes to resolve such things. In the fourteen years that I've been in practice it can be in as little as an hour depending upon the issue, how much you are invested in holding onto the idea and how ingrained it is.

Chapter 15) Yoga for Tension Headaches

Yoga can be a highly effective way for reducing the excess tension that can lead to head pain. Yoga will work to reduce tension headaches in many ways.

First, it will help to reduce the tension that accumulates in the shoulder and neck area which will help to prevent the muscles in the upper body area from contracting and causing a tension headache.

Practising yoga will also help to calm the mind, helping to ease tension, stress and anxiety and the tension headaches that can often come with stress.

People often find when they practise yoga, that they sleep much better and getting a good night's sleep will also enable people to feel much more able to cope with the day ahead, and yoga will enhance focus and concentration, too.

Yoga comes in many forms. Ashtanga yoga can be used to calm the mind as well as energising the body and improving muscle strength while other forms such as hatha yoga work at a much slower pace and are useful for unwinding.

Some prefer to practice yoga at the start of the day to prepare them for their busy schedule. However, it is extremely beneficial to practice in the evening when the body and mind need to relax after a long day.

Before practicing yoga, wear loose clothes, make sure that your surroundings are quiet and that you won't be disturbed and make sure that the room is not too hot or too cold.

Don't practice yoga directly after eating and leave about two hours after a large meal before beginning any type of yoga practice.

Note: Patients suffering from high blood pressure or patients prone to headaches or migraines should take medical advice before practising Downward Dog or any of the inverted postures.

1) Forward Bend

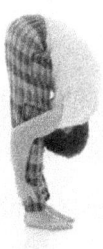

Forward bend poses help to calm and relax the mind so they can be practiced at any time when you feel the need to relax or when the mind feels as though it is racing.

Directions:

With an exhale, reach up with your hands above your head and on the inhale slowly come down. Reach your arms until they can hold your legs just above the ankle.

Hold the pose for five breaths and keep the breath smooth and relaxed. Exhale to come back up.

This pose also provides a strong stretch for the hamstrings and can help to loosen up a tight lower back.

For a gentler version of the above exercise, reach out to a chair instead of reaching all the way down.

Precautions:

Some people develop headaches when practising forward bend poses. However, this is usually caused by the alignment when in the pose and not by the pose itself.

Patients with blood pressure problems, hamstring problems or on-going headaches should seek advice before practising the move.

2) Child's Pose

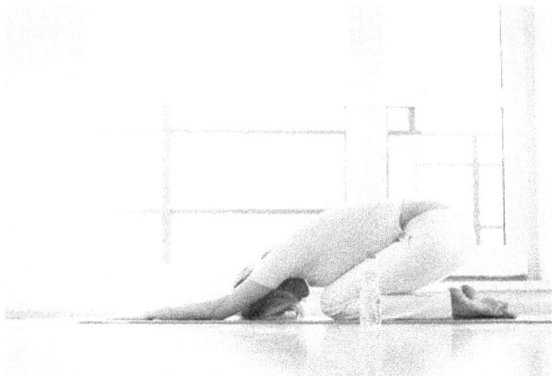

This posture is ideal for unwinding at the end of a long day. By stretching the hands forward, a deep stretch can be felt in the shoulder blades and the upper back.

Stretch your arms out as far as you comfortably can while in this position, and you'll get a much deeper stretch in the shoulder area.

Directions:

Kneel on a mat or soft surface and sit up straight. Exhale, and as you inhale fold forward so that the torso is rested on the chest and your arms are stretched out above your head.

Precautions:

People with lower back or knee problems and patients with high or low blood pressure should not practice this move.

3) Downward Dog Pose

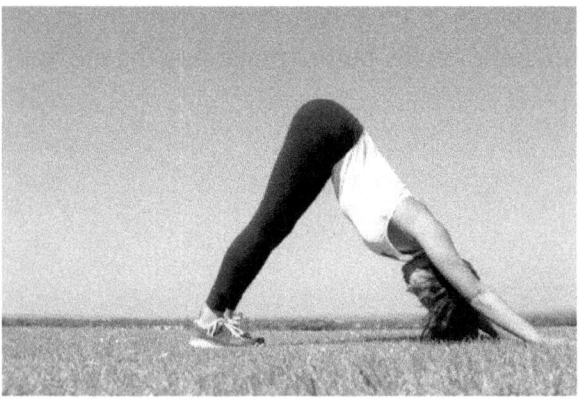

Downward Dog can be used on its own or as part of the Sun Salutation set of postures. The Downward Dog posture will stretch your shoulders and your chest, and will also help to calm your mind. It also helps to stretch the calves and Achilles tendon, so it is an ideal all over stretch if you are sat in one position all day.

You can get into this posture by kneeling, then reaching your hands forward, breathe out and gradually lift your knees. Press your hands firmly into the ground and continue to straighten your hands and knees until you reach the inverted V position.

To come out of this posture, gently lower your knees back to the floor.

Precautions:

Care should be taken not to lock the knees or the elbows while in this posture. Avoid this move if you have wrist, shoulder, arm, back or hip problems.

4) Seated Forward Bend © f9photos - Fotolia.com

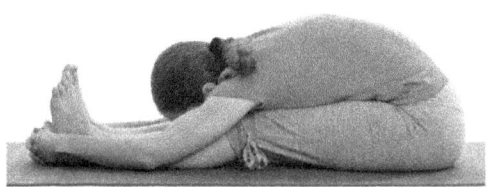

This yoga posture will also help to release tight back muscles and will help calm the mind after a long day.

Directions:

Sit up straight with both legs straight out in front of you. Inhale as you raise both arms until they are straight, then on the exhale lean forward and take hold of the soles of your feet with your hands. If you don't have enough flexibility to do this then use a yoga belt or an exercise band. Deepen the stretch by inhaling again and exhaling to relax further into the stretch. Hold the pose for up to thirty seconds. Inhale to come up.

Precautions:

This move should not be attempted if you have back, leg or shoulder problems.

Chapter 16) Vitamins, Minerals and Natural Products

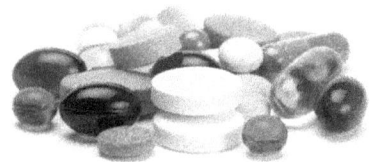

The products included in this chapter have been selected as they either help the body to manage stress and reduce anxiety, help to lift the mood, or can help to reduce pain in some patients.

The mood enhancing products will help reduce anxiety and leave people feeling like they are better able to cope with stress. However, if you are on medication for your headaches, on medication for stress, depression or anxiety, or are taking any other medication, then speak to your GP first in case there are any contraindications.

This chapter will also highlight some of the natural supplements that have been suggested to naturally treat depression and anxiety and detail some of the potential negative implications from taking them.

1) B Complex Vitamins

B complex vitamins can help the body to manage stress and when the body and mind is stressed, B complex vitamins tend to get used up more than they normally would. B vitamins help the adrenal glands to function properly and the adrenal glands need to function well in order to defeat stress. B vitamins are also essential to the health of the brain and the nervous system.

Taking a B complex supplement will help to keep stores of these vitamins from depleting when the body is under stress. Either take them in tablet form or buy a liquid supplement and add it to water. The liquid form is good to use during the day when feeling stressed as it will have an uplifting effect on the mood.

Add the liquid B complex to some water or orange juice and drink it when required, but do not exceed the stated amount.

2) Fish Oil/Omega 3

Fish oil has a mood enhancing effect and can help to lift the mood when a person is feeling moderately depressed. Fish should be eaten regularly for its mood enhancing qualities and the mind will often be much calmer after eating a meal containing fish as the uplifting effects of the omega 3 oils will help to banish anxiety and help to reduce the negative mind chatter that can occur when a person has a low mood.

Fish oil can also be bought as capsules or in a liquid form, but don't supplement with the oil or eat excessive amount of oily fish if you are on blood thinning medication.

Omega 3 can also be obtained from nuts and seeds, some vegetables and tofu.

3) Vitamin D

Not only is vitamin D essential for helping to build strong bones, it is also thought to help patients with mild depression. Vitamin D can be obtained from foods such as oily fish and dairy products. The richest source of vitamin D is from the natural sunlight.

Being out in the sunshine will help to lift the mood and aid relaxation as well.

4) Calcium

While the mineral magnesium helps the muscles to relax, calcium makes them contract. This might not sound like the obvious solution to people if they already have tight, tense muscles, however, some people do find that taking calcium can work for them.

However, there have been some health warnings over calcium supplementation in recent years and some people find that too much calcium can contribute to a headache.

5) SAMe

SAMe or S-adenosyl-l-methionine, which is a natural substance, has been shown to have mood lifting effects, and many believe that it could be a natural alternative to taking anti-depressants.

Studies have shown that the substance works better than a placebo and that results when taking it were comparable to tricyclic antidepressants. However, more research is needed into this.

SAMe is also believed to be an effective natural pain reliever, especially for patients with arthritis.

There are also some side effects that some people experience when taking SAMe as a supplement. The supplement shouldn't be taken by patients who are already on medication to increase their serotonin levels and it can increase anxiety levels in some patients. Other side effects can include insomnia and digestive problems.

This is a supplement that can be readily bought. However, it is not a supplement that should be taken without getting medical advice first.

6) Ginseng

Ginseng comes in various forms, including Siberian, Korean and Asian. The Siberian form of ginseng is an adaptogenic, meaning that it supports the adrenal glands and help the body to cope better with stress.

People often take ginseng during times of stress or heavy workloads as it can increase the stamina and leave a person feeling much more able to cope with the demands of their day. Some people also say that ginseng helps improve their concentration and the herb will make people feel more alert.

The herb should not be taken last thing at night or too late in the afternoon as it acts as a stimulant and can cause problems sleeping.

Ginseng can be brought as tablets or capsules, teas or tinctures.

7) 5HTP

5HTP, or L-5-hydroxytryptophan, enables the brain to make serotonin. When our serotonin levels are high we tend to not suffer from depression or anxiety or the emotional stress that contribute to a tension-type headache.

For this reason, 5HTP is often suggested as a natural treatment for patients with depression. However, studies have shown that there are some contraindications for using 5HTP as a supplement on its own. One of the main issues that studies have highlighted is that when supplements such as 5HTP are taken on their own, they can decrease the levels of dopamine, a neurotransmitter produced by the brain that makes us feel good.

Although many people do report an improvement in their symptoms of depression when taking this supplement, it is not something that should be tried if you are already on any other kind of medication, and it shouldn't be taken if you are on sort of medication that is designed to lift or stabilise your moods.

8) Rescue Remedy

Rescue Remedy consists of five of the Bach Flower Remedies that are believed to help people cope with stressful, demanding situations and helps to bring a calm and stability to the mind.

The remedy is useful to people who are finding that they are prone to panic attacks and it can be especially useful to help calm the nerves when facing a stressful event such as a presentation or job interview.

The remedy can be taken in water, used as a spray, chewing gum, or in pastille form. It can be carried with you and used at any time when you feel stressed or unable to cope with a situation.

9) Guarana

Guarana lifts the mood due to its caffeine content, and many people find that it makes them feel energised, focused and much less stressed, as it improves their capability to get tasks completed.

People who are trying to manage a busy work/social/family life sometimes take guarana as it gives them the energy to cope with the many demands of modern-day society. However, due to its caffeine content, it won't be suitable for everyone.

This herbal product can be brought as tea, tinctures, alternative coffee mixes, gums, bars and capsules.

Due to the stimulating effects of this product, it should not be used late afternoon or late evening, or it will cause insomnia.

Contraindications:

As caffeine can significantly increase the heart rate in some people, this product should not be taken in excess, and it shouldn't be taken without medical consultation.

Guarana could also interact with some medications such as MAOIs that are used to treat depression and other disorders, anti-coagulant/blood thinning drugs, lithium and asthma medications, and some antibiotics might also interact with guarana.

If you are on medication of any kind, don't try this product without talking to a doctor first.

10) Magnesium

Alison Wyndham of the Wyndham Centre suggests people suffering from tension headaches might find the mineral magnesium useful in treating tension headaches:

"Magnesium tones the blood vessels and scientists have linked certain types of headache with blood flow and pressure in the vessels. Magnesium also helps to prevent muscle spasms and cramps which could benefit tension headaches. Take it with B6 as it helps to increase the amount of magnesium the cells absorb."

11) Vitamin B2

B2 (Riboflavin) is another vitamin suggested for the treatment of headaches. Alison Wyndham explains:

"B2 has been known to reduce the frequency of headaches. It helps to boost energy production in the nerves."

12) GABA

GABA or gamma-aminobutyric acid is a neurotransmitter that has been shown to help improve the mood. It is often taken at night time to help aid sleep and promote relaxation. However, this product is also known to increase the production of growth hormones so it is not a supplement that people should be taking without getting advice first.

13) Tryptophan

Tryptophan is an amino acid that is known to lift the mood and also aids sleep. Tryptophan can be obtained from the diet or in supplement form. The chapter on mood foods details some of the foods that contain this amino acid.

Contraindications:

There are many drugs that can interact with tryptophan, especially anti-depressant medications and shouldn't be taken without medical advice.

14) Avena Sativa

Avena Sativa, or wild oats, is a well-known natural treatment for helping to reduce stress and anxiety.

Oats are rich in B vitamins, which means they can help the body to cope during stressful periods.

Avena Sativa can be taken as capsules, tinctures, and drops.

15) Skullcap

As well as being a relaxant, the herb can be an effective treatment for a headache, especially if the pain is caused by a contraction – or spasm – in the neck muscles.

The herb can be bought in capsule form, a tincture and as a dried herb. Some relaxing tea blends also contain skullcap as an ingredient due to its sedative effect.

Precautions:

Patients on anti-depressants or medications that have a sedative effect should not use skullcap. As with any of the other herbal or natural supplements listed in this book, if a patient is on any form of medication, they should discuss natural treatment options with their doctor first.

16) Vervain

Vervain is another herb that is known for its sedating, relaxant effects. It is good for use in the early evening or for last thing at night.

This herb is also one of the natural remedies for a headache and it can help reduce insomnia and anxiety.

It can be drunk as a tea, used as a tincture or taken as a herbal supplement.

Contraindications:

Patients already taking medication for a medical condition should take advice before using this herbal remedy.

Chapter 17) Relaxation Methods

Whenever there is tightness or tension in the body, then there will almost inevitably be pain. The following chapter examines the powerful techniques that can be used to relax the mind and the body and they will be helpful to patients who find stress is a trigger for a tension-type headache. The following techniques do not offer a cure for tension headaches, but by practicing regular relaxation techniques, a patient can reduce the amount of painful attacks.

1) Meditation

Meditation is a powerful form of relaxation and the techniques learned can be used at any moment of the day. Whether you are stressed at work, trying to juggle a busy family life, or simply find it hard to wind down, then meditation can help.

As well as helping people to manage stress, guided meditations can also be an excellent way to help headache sufferers to manage pain. In addition, regular practice of meditation can help to reduce high blood pressure and lower cortisol levels.

There are many free courses available online. Some websites have files to download so people can choose a meditation that suits their needs. Once the meditation technique has been perfected, then it can be called upon whenever you need it.

Meditations can also be downloaded as an app, which is good for people who have rushed lives and want something calming and relaxing as they go about their day.

2) Visualisation

Visualisation is often used to help people to set goals. Some people believe that by picturing themselves being successful they will then become successful. Visualisation could be used in the run up to a sports event or when preparing for a presentation at work. By picturing something going well, this automatically reduces stress and helps to allay anxiety in the run up to an event.

However, many people also use creative visualisation to help manage their health issues. For instance, if tension is an issue, a person can create a picture in their mind of becoming more relaxed, or if a person has a headache coming on, then they picture the pain easing.

Creative visualisation is about creating positive images that counter the stressful situations that a person might be facing and it is an effective way of creating a more positive mind-set.

3) Cognitive Behavioural Therapy

Cognitive Behavioural Therapy or Cognitive Behaviour Therapy (CBT) has become increasingly popular over the last few years to help patients suffering from depression, anxiety and stress.

CBT enables patients to learn healthy habits and attitudes that make everyday life much easier to cope with as well as helping patients to manage stressful situations more easily. There is a lot of evidence to support the effectiveness of CBT and this form of therapy is increasingly being used by counsellors to help people through difficult times in their lives.

If stress is one of the major causes of your tension headaches, then CBT could be one of the best options for you. Doctors in the UK can refer patients for this kind of treatment. However, as there is such a high demand for the service, the waiting lists are very long: four months or more in some places.

However, there are plenty of books and CDs on the subject of CBT and there are several courses that are available online to help patients who need help to manage stress.

4) Hypnosis/Self Hypnosis

Hypnosis is a powerful way to help patients combat any stress-related problems that they might be experiencing. It can be used for anything from defeating anxiety to managing weight loss. Although it can be expensive, it can be the preferred way for some people when it comes to overcoming mental blocks or stressful periods in their life.

Some patients aren't comfortable with the thought of not being in control of a situation and for this reason they might not consider using this form of therapy. However, there are self-hypnosis books and CDs available that are ideal for patients who want to try this type of therapy for themselves in the comfort of their own homes.

5) Tai Chi

The gentle, flowing movements that are a part of Tai Chi can have an extremely calming effect on the mind, helping to counter stress and anxiety and will also help to promote a feeling of well-being. In addition, Tai Chi can improve co-ordination, focus and concentration and help a person to feel more alert. The slow movements help to cultivate a sense of calmness so if you know that there is a stressful time coming up, then Tai Chi can help to better manage the stress.

This form of exercise is easy to follow, even for the beginner, and makes an ideal activity for winding down at the end of the long day. For people who don't want to join a class, then DVDs make a great alternative.

6) Stretching

Tension in the neck and shoulder area is a common cause of tension headaches. This can be a particular problem for people who spent a lot of time sitting in one position while at work or at home.

People who do a lot of computer work will find regular stretching beneficial and it can help to lessen the amount of tension headaches. Just gently turning the neck from side to side is a simple stretch that can be practiced while sitting at a desk or during a break. In addition, carefully tilting the head to one side until a stretch is felt in the neck is another good way to reduce tension in this area. Make sure to repeat the stretch on the other side too.

Remember to perform these stretches carefully and don't make any sudden or jerky moves as the neck area is extremely vulnerable to injury.

To stretch the shoulder, lean forward from a chair and gently swing the shoulder from side to side to loosen up the shoulder joint.

7) Affirmations

As with creative visualisation, affirmations are a popular way to help create a positive image in the mind, helping a person to feel more positive about a situation they are facing.

There is a simple idea behind using affirmations: rather than spending time worrying or fretting about an upcoming event or a difficulty, a person instead creates positive thoughts by using positive words and phrases.

Just thinking positively can help to create an entirely different outlook on life and on any problems that might lie ahead.

Chapter 18) Exercises for Tension Headaches

These exercises aren't aimed at relieving the headaches themselves. However, they do act as an effective remedy for a headache by reducing the tension in the shoulder and neck.

As you will have learned by now, muscle tension and headache go hand in hand. So in order to reduce the headaches, it is vital to find ways of effectively managing tension that has accumulated in the upper body area.

1) Shoulder Stretch

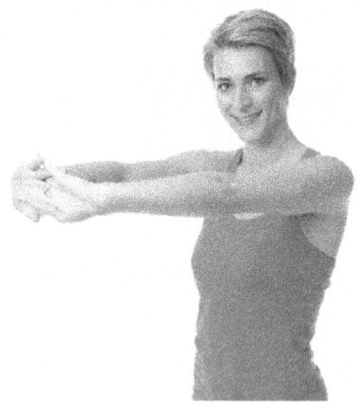

This exercise will help to relax the shoulders and the top of the back. It is especially useful for people who do a lot of computer work or sit in one position for long periods of time.

The stretch can be carried out throughout the day and it will help to release the tightness that starts to build in the neck muscles as well.

Don't wait for your shoulders to begin to feel tight. Instead, stretch them out throughout the day to prevent tension from building up in the upper body area in the first place.

Directions:

Interlink the fingers and stretch them out. As you relax into the stretch, curl your neck forward slightly to enhance the stretch in the shoulder area. This stretch will also be felt in the back of the neck.

The stretch should be held for 15-30 seconds and repeated 2-3 times. Office workers can benefit from doing this stretch as often as possible, and it is beneficial for occupations such as hairdressing as well.

2) Shoulder Exercise

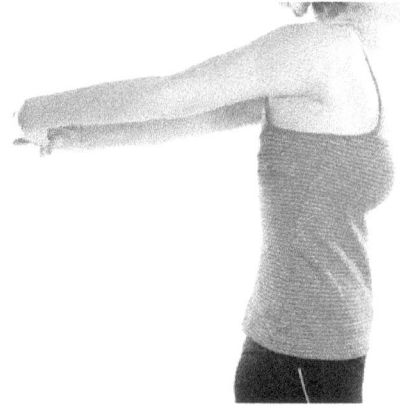

The following exercise will help to reduce tension in the shoulder area as well as opening up the chest.

Directions:

Interlink your fingers behind you and then gently stretch your arms upwards. Hold until you feel a stretch in the shoulder and chest area.

The position should be held for 15-30 seconds and repeated three times.

3) Shoulder Stretch Three

This is a good exercise to assess just how much tightness and flexibility there is in the shoulder area. The aim is to be able to interlink both hands on both sides. However, many people will find that the range of motion in the shoulder area is either so limited that they can make both fingers reach, or they'll find that they can complete the stretch on one side but not on the other.

Some people might also find that they can do the stretch one day but not the next. This is due to the muscles being tighter some days than they are others.

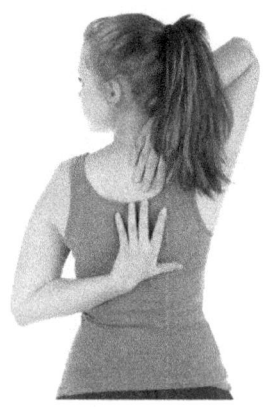

Directions:

Walk the fingers of your right hand down towards the middle of your upper back. Bring the fingers of the left hand behind you and then reach them up to so the fingertips of the left hand touch the fingertips of the right hand.

Don't force this movement and, if you cannot connect both hands, just stretch as far as you can or use a belt or exercise band.

4) Neck Stretch on a Ball

This exercise is especially good for excessive tightness in the neck region. It is performed lying down and the ball provides some resistance to stretch out against. Because of this, the stretch is more effective. However, it can also feel more intense so this exercise should be stopped the moment any discomfort is felt.

This exercise should be performed lying down.

Place a ball under the neck: a medium sized ball with medium resistance is ideal for this. Gently turn the neck all the way to the left, hold for a few seconds, and then return to the centre.

To complete the stretch, turn the neck to the right and hold for as long as is comfortable. This exercise can be repeated for a maximum of ten times, but start with small, gentle repetitions until the worst of the tension has been eased out.

The exercise can be repeated three to five times on both sides and can be done throughout the day to reduce and prevent tension from building up.

Chapter 19) Feeling Good

Avoiding tension headaches means finding ways to keep yourself feeling good and the mood elevated. When the mood is lifted, people don't tend to worry or stress about things so much. Medication isn't always required to keep the mood elevated. Here are some methods to help produce a natural high.

1) The Importance of Exercise

Exercise is important for the production of a hormone called serotonin. This is the hormone that is produced by the body naturally and allows us to feel good. However, some people have low levels of serotonin, which can leave them feeling stressed, anxious, or unable to cope. This kind of emotional stress is one of the causes of tension headaches, so finding a form of exercise that you enjoy can be an important tool for managing tension type headaches.

Exercise is also excellent for maintaining a healthy weight, keeping the heart in good condition and promoting circulation. In addition, exercise also helps a person to sleep better and a good night's sleep will leave you feeling more able to manage stress and cope with the day ahead.

Obviously, you shouldn't be exercising if you are feeling at all unwell and the forms of exercise detailed here should be seen as a preventative measure more than anything else.

Experts say that in order to get enough exercise, we should find an activity we enjoy and exercise for at least 30 minutes five times a week.

a) Walking

Walking outside in the fresh air is an effective way to help beat stress. Sometimes just getting some time out of the home, office, or out of a stressful situation can make all the difference and give you the opportunity to find some perspective in the stresses that you might be feeling.

b) Exercise Classes

Exercises classes aren't for everyone, but they make a great social activity and many people find them uplifting. It doesn't have to be anything too jarring on the joints such as an aerobics class, but something low impact is ideal. Some people find that dance classes will lift their mood and help them feel energized, while others prefer something more relaxing such as a stretch class or Tai Chi.

c) Exercise DVDs

If you really can't face a fitness class, but still want to get the benefits from regular exercise, then fitness DVDs are a good option. Whether it is a low impact aerobics class, or a simple yoga routine, you can find something simple and enjoyable that will help you to increase your serotonin levels,

If you haven't exercised for a while, try some of the beginner videos and stick to large floor based exercise routines so that you don't put too much stress on the joints. Avoid anything that suggests jerky movements as this can increase the tension and tightness in the shoulder area.

2) Run a Bath

There are few things more relaxing that sitting back in a hot bath. Not only does this have a positive effect on the body by allowing the muscles to relax, it also helps the mind to unwind as well.

Taking a long, relaxing bath before bed is one of the ways to help ensure a good night's sleep. Use some relaxing bath oils or add some essential oils such as lavender, ylang ylang or chamomile.

3) Enjoy Yourself

When we are busy, we have much less time to worry about other things. Engaging in a hobby – whether it is alone or with a group of people – is an ideal therapy for forgetting about any stresses and tensions for a while and concentrating on something else.

Creative hobbies such as arts and crafts are especially effective at helping a person to relax and unwind.

And take time out to laugh more. Whether it is watching a favourite comedy or having a talk with friends, these are all things that will lift the mood and help to curb anxiety and worry, thus helping to manage some of the emotional stress that can trigger a tension-type headache.

4) SAD Therapy

During the long, winter nights and the dark winter mornings, many people find themselves feeling depressed. This is referred to as SAD or Seasonal Affective Disorder. The lack of sunshine during the winter months can mean that the serotonin levels dip, leaving people depressed, and along with depression comes the feeling of not being able to cope with stress or feelings of anxiety.

One way of preventing SAD is to get a lightbox. These provide an artificial light that has been designed to act as artificial sunlight, thus boosting the mood during the dark days and nights of winter.

5) Natural Alarm Clocks

When it's cold outside, people often start to feel sluggish and this can sometimes mean sleeping in later than usual and not getting everything done on time. This can be mean a lot of rushing around at the last minute to get things done, causing the mind and body yet more stress.

Natural alarm clocks can help ease the sluggish feeling by helping a person to wake up gradually and help to keep a sense of well-being all day long.

This will mean being less stressed as a person goes about their daily activities and will help in getting up at the same time every day. Getting up at the same time every day is essential for a healthy body clock.

6) Listen to Music

Listening to music can be elevating for the mood. Most people will have had a moment when they've been feeling down and then a song has come on the radio that has lifted their mood and helped them to feel better about things.

Music has been used as therapy for a long time and there are CD compilations that have been designed specifically to help a person manage stress.

Music can also be used to help reduce anxiety.

Chapter 20) Mood Foods and Diet

Eating the right kinds of foods can help keep our moods lifted. When the mood is even, people are much less likely to worry about things or have anxieties that constantly distract them. For this reason, eating the right kinds of foods can help prevent tension-type headaches by helping to prevent the stressed feeling that contributes to them.

Certain foods can help level out our serotonin levels and, as explained earlier in the book, serotonin is what makes us feel good.

If you often feel stressed, angry, or have a low mood after a meal, then look at your diet and modify it. Look at ways that you can add more serotonin rich foods to your diet and include them every day, especially during stressful times.

Detailed below are some of the foods that can help increase levels of serotonin.

1) Potatoes

Potatoes are known to increase the serotonin levels. Having a baked potato at lunchtime can help to keep the mood lifted throughout the afternoon and will help a person to feel less stressed.

As potatoes can give quite a sharp rise in the blood sugar levels, they are best eaten with a serving of protein such as cheese, tuna, baked beans etc.

2) Brown Rice

Brown rice will give the body a steady stream of energy and contains high levels of B vitamins that are essential for keeping the mood steady and helping the body to feel energized.

Complex carbohydrates such as brown rice will also keep the blood sugars even, and a steady blood sugar will help to ease anxiety and stress.

3) Poultry

White meats such as turkey and chicken contain tryptophan, the amino acid that is essential for the production of serotonin. Meats such as chicken and turkey are also low in fat, so they are much healthier to eat on a regular basis than red meat.

4) Cottage Cheese

Dairy foods also contain tryptophan and should be included in the diet regularly. If you are concerned about fat levels, then go for the lighter versions of dairy products or try cottage cheese, which is low in fat.

5) Beans and Pulses

Legumes are a low glycaemic food, which means they won't cause a surge in the blood sugar level after you have eaten them. This is important because when the glucose levels surge it can cause cortisol levels to rise, adding to stress levels.

Beans and pulses might not seem appealing to some people and some of them can be a little bland, however, legumes are also extremely versatile and they can be used in a vast array of recipes including curries, casseroles, salads and soups.

6) Nuts and Seeds

Nuts and seeds are an excellent way to keep serotonin levels boosted throughout the day. They are great for snacks in the mid-afternoon and evening when the blood sugar often dips.

Seeds and nuts can be scattered over salads, on breakfast cereals and toast or they can be eaten alongside a carbohydrate snack to help keep the blood sugar levels steady throughout the day.

7) Keeping the Blood Sugar Levels Steady

When the blood sugar is out of control, the mind and body will be under a great deal of stress. Glucose levels that swing from high to low will lead to low moods and unbalanced hormone levels, As a result, low blood sugars will lead to the body producing cortisol, leaving a person feeling stressed and anxious.

When the blood sugars are out of control, people are more prone to headaches and the low moods that come with poorly controlled glucose levels will cause anxiety and feelings of depression. For this reason, a good diet is key to keeping yourself feeling good.

The answer to ending the blood sugar rollercoaster is to eat complex carbohydrates that give the body a consistent source of energy, rather than foods that turn into sugar too quickly and cause the blood sugar to spike after a meal.

One of the best ways to keep the blood sugar steady throughout the day is to eat little and often. Three balanced meals and three small snacks between meals are better than eating three large meals a day.

Main meals should be based on complex carbohydrates such as granary bread, wholemeal or basmati rice, wholemeal pastas, lentils, pulses and grains such as barley, bulgur wheat and quinoa.

Breakfasts should consist of slow burning carbohydrates such as oatmeal, porridge or muesli – choose the no added sugar variety – with a serving of protein such as a boiled egg.

Mid-morning and afternoon snacks should consist of fruit, oatcakes, or anything that will give a constant supply of glucose. Fruit shouldn't be eaten on their own as some people find that even the naturally occurring sugars in fruit can be enough to cause their blood sugar to soar, especially if their glucose levels are already imbalanced. Instead, eat fruit with nuts or seeds.

If you are going to eat chocolate or something else sweet, then the best time to do this is with your main meal. By doing this, it will help to curb any surge in the blood sugar levels. In addition, adding ingredients such as cider vinegar or cinnamon to a meal will help to improve the blood sugar levels after a meal.

Finally, learn to look out for added sugar that is often included in some snacks and ready meals. Many shop bought products can look healthy, but on closer inspection they often contain an array of different types of sugars.

Appendix One: Balm Recipe

One small tin (lip balm size or slightly larger) for storage

One small bar of cosmetic beeswax

3-5 drops of vitamin E to act as a preservative

Essential Oils of your choice (choose from Ylang Ylang, chamomile, lavender, peppermint, rosemary, wintergreen or any essential oil that makes you feel relaxed or that lifts your mood.

Directions:

Using a double boiler, add some water in the bottom pan and gently heat the beeswax in the top part.

Once the beeswax has melted, stir in the vitamin E oil. Remove the mixture from the heat and then add 8-10 drops of your chosen essential oils.

Mix the oils in well with a spatula and then pour in to a storage jar. (Be careful not to get the mixture anywhere near your hands as it will be scalding hot)

Leave the jar in its place as it will be too hot to touch and leave the mixture to go solid and to cool down. It is best left overnight.

Apply the mixture whenever you feel a tension headache starting or put on the pulse points of the wrist and the neck during the day to help maintain a feeling of well-being.

Appendix Two: Seated Relaxation

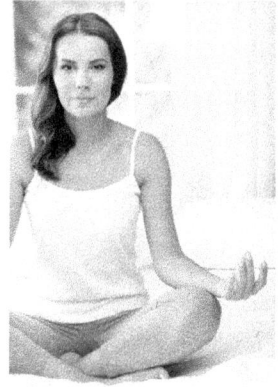

Everyone needs to take time out to relax. Whenever you feel yourself getting stressed or anxious or when you know that there is a stressful period coming, take a few minutes out to relax and centre yourself.

Learning to relax will help aid concentration and focus and can often help you to look at a situation in a different way. Whenever you feel the need, follow this seated relaxation and take some time out for yourself.

Directions:

Begin by sitting in a cross legged position. If this isn't comfortable, try sitting up straight on a chair.

Next, either rest your hands in your lap if you are seated or sit with your fingers as pictured above if you are in the cross legged pose. If you find this uncomfortable after a while, then place your hands on your knees.

Close your eyes and begin to count your breath until it slows. It might take a few moments to calm your mind and you might find distracting thoughts keep occurring, but the more you learn to relax the less this will happen.

Once your breath is calm and steady, stay in the same position with your eyes closed for at least five to ten minutes, until you find that your mind starts to relax and you feel revived and focused.

This pose is good for last thing at night to unwind before bed and it is ideal for starting the day with a feeling of calmness, especially if you have a long day ahead.

Appendix Three: Deep Relaxation

This relaxation is ideal for doing last thing at night. It will help to unwind the mind and body before sleep and reduce any tension that might have accumulated throughout the body during the day. It will also calm the mind and help aid a better night's sleep. After practicing the deep relaxation for a while, you should begin to feel more rested when you wake up the next morning.

Directions:

Lie back on the bed. The room should be comfortably warm and ideally the light should be dim.

Begin by counting back from twenty until the muscles begin to feel as though they are relaxing. If your mind is tense, begin to calm it down by thinking relaxing thoughts or repeat some affirmations until you find that any stresses or concerns start to ease.

Next, scrunch your toes as tight as you can, hold them for a few seconds and then relax.

Circle your ankles five times to the left and then five times to the right; tense the ankle joint gently and then relax it.

Continue the tensing and relaxation of each part of your lower body.

When you have finished relaxing each part of the lower body, then begin to concentrate on the upper body. Circle the wrists five times clockwise and five times anti-clockwise, then create a fist with each hand, hold for five seconds and then relax.

Do the same with each muscle in the upper body area and concentrate on the head and neck area, where tension tends to gather.

Using gentle, controlled movements, move your neck to the left, and then slowly to the right. Repeat this three to five times on each side.

Once you have tensed and relaxed all of your muscles, take a few moments to relax further. Perhaps use some of the meditation techniques or a visualisation exercise to help increase the feelings of relaxation.

Before starting the deep relaxation, you can also do a few stretches to help reduce excess tension.

Further Reading

Cluster Headaches: Treatment and Relief for Cluster, Cluster Migraine, and Recurring Eye-stab Pain, Goldstein, Michael

Cluster Headaches: Causes, Tests, and Treatment Options, Glenn, Jeremy, MA and Garfield, M.D, Arnold.

Headache: A Pratical Manual, Kernick, David and Goadsby, Peter J.

Coping with Headaches and Migraine, Frith, Alison

Change Your Thinking with CBT: Overcome Stress, Combat Anxiety and Improve Your Life, Edelmen, Dr, Sarah

Mind Over Mood: Change How You Feel By Changing the Way You Think, Aaron, Beck T., Greenberger, Dennis, Padesky, Christine A

Heal your Headache, Buchholz, David and Reich, Stephen G.

DVDs

Yoga for Health: Headaches with Jenny Cornero

Yoga for Health: Basics and Headaches

Tai Chi for Beginners

CDs

Guided Meditations for Stress Reduction, Bodhipaska

Creative Visualization, Gawain, Shakti

Suppliers

The essential oils, vitamins, minerals and amino acids can all be obtained from health food stores. They can also be brought from specialist stores online. Some manufacturers also allow customers to buy products direct from their websites.

If there are any problems obtaining any of the products, then they can be purchased through stores like Amazon, who stock a large range of health products or on eBay, which can be cheaper depending on where you are located.

The herbal products mentioned are available in tablets, tinctures and teas and can be brought from health stores offline or from specialist stores online.

Ice packs and heat packs can be obtained from sports stores.

To find an alternative practitioner such as an acupuncturist, an aromatherapist or an osteopath, there are several online directories that can be searched via postcode or zip code to find the one nearest to you.

All of the books, CDs and DVDs can be obtained online through stores like Amazon or through specialist book stores.

If there are any problems obtaining any of the products detailed in the book then contact the manufacturers or publishers for a list of suppliers.

Forums

Forums are useful for sharing personal experiences and for getting tips and advice from sufferers of cluster headaches and tension type headaches. The forums are all welcoming places to be and sharing your symptoms with someone else who understands them can be an important lifeline for many people suffering from head pain.

There are plenty of threads where people share advice on headache cures, headache relief and natural remedies for headaches. Alternatively, if anyone has an effective headache remedy or headache treatment that they would like to share, then they can start their own threads.

Listed below are some of the forums and support groups that can be found online.

Clusterheadaches.com

This is a support site that has been set up specifically for people who suffer from cluster headaches and also for the people who support them.

The site is packed full of useful information for cluster headache sufferers and also has a message board, quizzes and surveys as well as a selection of other features.

In order to contribute to the site, people have to register first. A good place to start is the new visitors' page that will take new users through all of the aspects of the site:

http://www.clusterheadaches.com/

The Cluster Headache Support Group

As well as detailing the symptoms and support that is available to cluster headache sufferers, the site also has a place where people can discuss their symptoms and the option of creating a cluster headache diary so people can record their attacks along with possible triggers.

In the forum, people can discuss anything related to cluster headaches such as how to find cluster headache relief, causes of headache, chronic cluster headaches, the treatment of cluster headaches, headache and pain relief, the cause of cluster headaches as well as home remedies for cluster headaches that patients might have found helpful for managing their symptoms.

http://www.clusterheadacheinfo.org/

OUCHUK

This is a UK-based charity that aims to support and raise awareness of cluster headaches. They have a forum as well, so people can connect with other people who understand their symptoms.

People can discuss their cluster headache symptoms, different types of cluster headache treatment, how to cope with cluster headache symptoms, cluster headaches causes etc.

The site can be found at: https://ouchuk.org/

Health Central

Although this forum concentrates mainly on migraines, there are a number of threads on tension headaches and people with long term head pain. On the forum, people can share their experiences of medications, physicians, alternative therapies, remedies for headaches, tension headache relief and tips on how to stop headaches.

http://forums.healthcentral.com

eHealthforum

The site has a forum where people can detail their symptoms of head pain. The community is very supportive and if there are questions that you haven't had the chance to ask a doctor, or if you just want to find someone to talk to, then there are plenty of opportunities to join in conversations or to start your own thread.

There is plenty of opportunity to discuss experiences of chronic headache, chronic tension headaches, cures for headaches, experiences of chronic daily headache and natural headache relief.

http://ehealthforum.com

Medhelp.org

When it comes to learning how to deal with tension headaches, there are plenty of helpful forums on the Internet, and Medhelp.org is one of them.

There are several discussions on this site about managing symptoms and people with chronic or episodic tension headaches share their experiences and answer questions where they can.

Members can also discuss how to alleviate tension headaches, treatment for tension headaches and what causes tension headaches.

Visitors can also share the latest news in chronic tension headache relief and tension headache treatments as well as share information on tension headache cures and the most effective tension headache medication.

http://www.medhelp.org

Acknowledgements

Thank you to Tim Allardyce from Croydon Physio

Val from the Organisation for the Understanding of Cluster Headaches

Alison Wyndham from the Wyndham Centre

Linda Southall from the Holistic Centre for Aromatherapy and Wellbeing

Marilyn Devonish from Trance Formations

And the staff at the Acumedic Clinic for their explanations of Chinese Medicine and acupuncture. Special Thanks to:

Christopher Delage

Julian Yates

Richard Eason

Published by IMB Publishing 2014

Index